KEY TOPICS IN

# CLINICAL RESEARCH

## A user guide to researching, analyzing and publishing clinical data

**F Gao Smith**
MB, BS, FRCA, MPhil
*Consultant in Anaesthesia and Intensive Care Medicine,*
*Birmingham Heartlands Hospital,*
*Birmingham, UK*

**J E Smith**
MB, ChB, FRCA
*Consultant in Anaesthesia and Intensive Care Medicine,*
*University Hospital Birmingham,*
*Selly Oak Hospital, Birmingham, UK*

BIOS

© BIOS Scientific Publishers Limited, 2003

First published 2003

A CIP catalogue record for this book is available from the British Library.

ISBN 1 85996 028 6

BIOS Scientific Publishers Ltd
9 Newtec Place, Magdalen Road, Oxford OX4 1RE, UK
Tel. +44 (0)1865 726286. Fax +44 (0)1865 246823
World Wide Web home page: http://www.bios.co.uk/

Distributed exclusively in the United States, its dependent territories, Canada, Mexico, Central and South America, and the Caribbean by Springer-Verlag New York Inc., 175 Fifth Avenue, New York, USA, by arrangement with BIOS Scientific Publishers Ltd., 9 Newtec Place, Magdalen Road, Oxford, OX4 1RE, UK

**Important Note from the Publisher**
The information contained within this book was obtained by BIOS Scientific Publishers Ltd from sources believed by us to be reliable. However, while every effort has been made to ensure its accuracy, no responsibility for loss or injury whatsoever occasioned to any person acting or refraining from action as a result of information contained herein can be accepted by the authors or publishers.

The reader should remember that medicine is a constantly evolving science and while the authors and publishers have ensured that all dosages, applications and practices are based on current indications, there may be specific practices which differ between communities. You should always follow the guidelines laid down by the manufacturers of specific products and the relevant authorities in the country in which you are practising.

Production Editor: Andrew Watts
Typeset by Servis Filmsetting Ltd, Manchester, UK
Printed by The Cromwell Press, Trowbridge, UK

# CONTENTS

# CONTRIBUTORS

**Lesley Allen BA (Hons)**
*Library Manager, Birmingham Heartlands Hospital, Birmingham, UK*

**Tar-Ching Aw PhD FFOM FRCPC FRCP FFPHM**
*Professor of Occupational Medicine, University of Kent at Canterbury, Kent, UK*

**Alan Casson MSc FRCSC FACS**
*Professor of Surgery, Head of Division of Thoracic Surgery, Dalhousie University and the QE II Health Science Centre, Nova Scotia, Canada*

**Somnath Chatterjee MD FRCA**
*Research Follow in Anaesthesia, Birmingham Heartlands Hospital, Birmingham, UK*

**Jonathan Cook BSc (Hons)**
*PhD student in Statistics, Health Services Research Unit, University of Aberdeen, Aberdeen, UK*

**Taj Dhallu FRCA**
*Consultant Anaesthetist, University Hospital of Wales, Cardiff, UK*

**Liam Lynch FFARCSI**
*Consultant Anaesthetist, Bon Secours Hospital, Tralee, Ireland*

**Craig Jackson MSc PhD**
*Senior Lecturer in Health Psychology, Facility of Health and Community Care, University of Central England, Birmingham, UK*

**Michael Kuo FRCS PhD DCH**
*Consultant Otolaryngologist – Head and Neck Surgeon, Birmingham Children's Hospital, Birmingham, UK*

**Daqing Ma MSc PhD**
*Research Associate, Imperial College School of Medicine, London, UK*

**Marcelle MacNamara FRCS MPhil**
*Consultant in Otolaryngologist – Head and Neck Surgeon, Birmingham Heartlands Hospital, Birmingham, UK*

**Graeme MacLennan BSc (Hons), PGCE**
*Statistician, Health Services Research Unit, University of Aberdeen, Aberdeen, UK*

**Danny McAuley MD MRCP DICM**
*SpR Respiratory Medicine and advanced level trainee Intensive Care Medicine, Birmingham Heartlands Hospital, Birmingham, UK*

**Magnus McGee BSc MSc**
*Senior Statistician, Health Services Research Unit, University of Aberdeen, Aberdeen, UK*

**Gavin Perkins MRCP FIMC RCS**
*Research Fellow in Intensive Care Medicine, Birmingham Heartlands Hospital, Birmingham, UK*

**Craig Ramsey Bsc PGDip PhD**
*Senior Statistician, Health Services Research Unit, University of Aberdeen, Aberdeen, UK*

**Sukhbinder Singh MRCP & FRCA**
*Clinical Research Fellow, Heart Hospital, London, UK*

**Richard Steyn FRCSEd (C-Th) MRCGP FIMC RCS MSc**
*Consultant in Thoracic Surgery, Birmingham Heartlands Hospital, Birmingham, UK*

**Michael Vickers FRCA**
*Professor Emeritus in Anaesthesia and Intensive Care Medicine, University of Wales College of Medicine, Cardiff, UK*

**Martin Wildman MRCP**
*MRC Training Fellow in Health Services Research, Department of Public Health and Policy, London School of Hygiene and Tropical Medicine, London, UK*

**Yinhua Zhang PhD**
*Lecturer in Physiology, University of Bristol, Bristol, UK*

# ABBREVIATIONS

| | |
|---|---|
| A&E | accident and emergency |
| ACE | angiotensin converting enzyme |
| ALA | allergy to laboratory animals |
| ANOVA | analysis of variance |
| APACHE | acute physiology and chronic health evaluation |
| BMJ | British Medical Journal |
| CABG | coronary artery bypass grafting |
| CINAHL | cumulative index of nursing and allied health literature |
| CME | continuing medical education |
| COPD | chronic obstructive pulmonary disease |
| CPD | continuing professional development |
| CPR | cardiopulmonary resuscitation |
| CV | coefficient of variation |
| DVR | data validation report |
| HIV | human immunodeficiency virus |
| ICNARC | intensive care national audit and research centre |
| ICU | intensive care unit |
| IVF | in vitro fertilization |
| LREC | local research ethics committee |
| LSD | least significant difference |
| MAP | mean arterial pressure |
| MCQ | multiple choice questions |
| MD | doctorate of medicine |
| MeSH | medical subject headings |
| MPM | mortality prediction models |
| MREC | multi-centre research ethics committee |
| NELH | National Electronic Library for Health |
| NHS | National Health Service |
| NLM | National Library of Medicine |
| NPV | negative predictive value |
| NYHA | New York Heart Association |
| OMNI | online medical networked information |
| OR | odds ratio |
| PEF | peak expiratory flow |
| PI | prediction interval |

PNA       phrenic nerve activity
PPV       positive predictive value
PRISM     paediatric risk of mortality
RCT       randomized controlled trials
ROC       receiver operating characteristic
RPCCT     randomised, prospective, controlled clinical trial
SAPS      simplified acute physiology score
$SaO_2$   arterial oxygen saturation
SD        standard deviation
SEM       standard error of the mean
SMR       standardized mortality ratio
$SpO_2$   pulse oxygen saturation
TRISS     trauma injury severity score
URTI      upper respiratory tract infection
www       world wide web

# PREFACE

There are many books designed to help postgraduate trainees undertake clinical audit and research projects. Other books help them to analyze their results using medical statistics. Yet more texts help them prepare for their specialty examinations. These books are often written by eminent senior researchers or statisticians and, unfortunately, to the hard-pressed medical trainee they may appear turgid, difficult to read and of tedious length. The idea for this book arose from a series of tutorials and courses given by the authors, who are clinical practitioners with special interests in clinical research, working at teaching hospitals. There is a continuing demand for a short, clear, highlighted reference to guide trainees and trainers through research and audit projects, from first idea, through data collection and analysis, to presentation and publication. The aim of this book is also to provide comprehensive, concise and easily accessible information on all aspects of research and audit for the busy young trainee preparing for his specialty examinations.

We are most grateful for the enthusiasm that all authors have brought to this venture, for the expert help of Professor MD Vickers in reviewing selected topics, and for the encouragement and patience of Ms Lisa Mansell at BIOS Scientific Publishers.

*Fang Gao Smith*
*John Eric Smith*

# MEDICAL RESEARCH AS PART OF POSTGRADUATE TRAINING

*Danny McAuley*

Most doctors planning to take part in research will not have had previous research experience. The decision to undertake research should be given proper consideration, because engaging in a research project will be time consuming, may influence career progression and may form the basis of a career-long research interest.

## Difference between medical research and clinical practice

The key difference is their scope. In each, information (data) is collected from individual subjects, but in medical research the aim is to be able to make some general statements about a wider set of subjects, and the researchers are not usually specifically interested in the particular subjects that have been studied. The subjects who are studied act as a proxy for the total group of interest. Researchers thus use information from a **sample** of individuals to make some **inference** about the wider **population** of like individuals, since researchers can never study, for example, all asthmatic patients.

## Benefits of undertaking medical research

- Scientific interest.
- Contribution to medical knowledge.
- Understanding research and statistical methods.
- Development of information technology skills.
- Ability to critically appraise a research paper.
- Career advancement through publication and obtaining a research degree.
- Identify if suited to academic career.

## When to undertake medical research

Currently, the majority of doctors undertake research during post-graduate training to allow career advancement.

*1.  Prior to specialist training.* Doctors may participate in research in order to obtain an appointment to a Specialist Registrar training programme. As a result, research is undertaken prior to gaining knowledge of one's planned area of specialization and the research fellow has only a limited idea of what is important and what they might find interesting.

*2.  During or after specialist training.* Alternatively, doctors may delay engaging in research until 2–3 years after starting a Specialist Registrar training programme. They will then have acquired an area of interest within their speciality and are more likely to develop a project in which they are intellectually engaged.

Unfortunately, requirements for entry into specialist medical training frequently remove the choice of when to do research. The time taken to develop a research project can not be over-estimated and, accordingly, plans to undertake a research project should begin well in advance of the anticipated starting date. How this period of research will be viewed in post-graduate specialist training can be gauged by discussion with the speciality advisor. With the agreement of the postgraduate dean and the speciality advisor, trainees may spend up to 3 years in research while retaining their national training number. Up to a year can contribute to the attainment of a certificate of completion of specialist training.

## Determining the research area

If the aim is simply career advancement then undertaking a designated project in the department of one's likely future area of specialization may be appropriate. But if the aim is to develop an understanding of the research process it is more appropriate to discuss common ideas of interest with the proposed supervisor and subsequently develop a protocol.

*1. The area of specialization.* The introduction of 'Calman' training, during which junior doctors are appointed to a speciality training scheme, has largely limited potential research areas to the likely area of specialization.

(a) *Potential advantages*
- One's clinical area of interest will match one's research area of interest.
- Communication at scientific meetings allows interaction with other workers in the same speciality.
- It allows the development of a career-long research interest within one's own speciality.

(b) *Potential disadvantages*
- There may be pressure to undertake medical research in a particular area: trainees may undertake research in which they may not be interested but which they recognize as a requirement for career advancement because it is ongoing in a department.
- If a trainee simply undertakes a project currently ongoing in a department as a technician, the important concepts of how to develop a research idea and develop and write a protocol will not be achieved.
- Lack of ownership of the project will potentially dampen long-term enthusiasm for medical research.

*2. The area of one's own interest.*

(a) *Advantages*
- It is likely that this approach will be associated with a more satisfying research experience.
- The research project can still be undertaken in the department of one's likely future area of specialization and will still have the benefits of career advancement. Ownership of the project generates greater enthusiasm and the researcher is likely to be more productive: this results in greater benefits for both researcher, in terms of career advancement, and for the department in which the research is undertaken.

## Ideal features of a department in which to undertake medical research

It is important to undertake the research project in an established department supervised by an active and productive researcher. A proven track record is likely to mean that the supervisor and the department are adequately funded and have the infrastructure to support research.

It should also be able to provide two types of supervisor: a clinical supervisor to help identify and develop the research project and a non-clinical scientist to establish laboratory-based work and to train in actual research skills and statistical methods.

1.  ***Experienced supervisors.*** These will be able to determine what can reasonably be expected to be completed within the given period. More importantly, if unforeseen difficulties arise they are likely to be able to provide timely advice regarding alternative strategies or projects.

2.  ***A track record of graduates achieving higher degrees and other research fellows working in the department.*** Research fellows will have the practical knowledge and time:

- To answer queries which arise almost daily, particularly at the start of the project.
- To exchange their experience and advice.
- To collaborate with each other on such matters as patient recruitment.

3.  ***Established techniques.*** Whilst not essential, it is certainly useful if the techniques which are to be used are established within the department in which you plan to work.

Although it is possible to apply a new technique to an area of research, there are potential problems. There will be no-one available to give practical advice on managing problems arising with the technique; novel techniques may have not been validated before.

4.  ***How to find out these requirements.***

- Medline searches for recent publications will determine if potential supervisors are active and productive.
- Grant success is a useful marker of the success of a department and a potential supervisor. This information can usually be obtained from individual medical schools.
- Previous and current research fellows can provide invaluable advice on these areas and, more importantly, they can provide information not available elsewhere regarding the support, encouragement and research training provided within the department overall.

5.  ***Go to meet the supervisor.*** It is important to approach your potential supervisor to discuss the possibility of undertaking research in his or her department. It is likely the potential supervisor will wish to see your curriculum vitae.

## Deciding whether to undertake an MD or a PhD

1.  ***Characteristics of an MD degree.*** Unless there are exceptional circumstances an MD can only be taken in the university which awarded the basic medical degree. The regulations vary widely between universities and it is essential to check on the requirements of your own university.

- An MD is characteristically less supervised, which can result in unfocused research.

- It is more usually funded by non-grant-giving bodies such as pharmaceutical companies and therefore the project may not have been subject to independent peer review.
- An MD can require a minimum of 2 years of research, although it is not unusual for a longer period of research to be undertaken.
- Although an MD may be undertaken on a part-time basis it is common for the majority of the research to be undertaken on a full time basis. There may be competing commitments with time divided between pharmaceutical trial work and the thesis.
- An MD more frequently involves clinical research and clinical commitment.
- In some universities it may be based on work already published.

2. *Characteristics of a PhD degree.* A PhD degree is based upon clearly defined research proposals and is usually more focused, with pre-agreed aims and subsequent close supervision.

- Research training fellowships supported by medical charities are more likely to be awarded for PhD study because of the perception that a PhD gives a better training in research methodology.
- The normal duration is 3 years but there is a trend for a PhD to last for 4 years, allowing students to undertake more detailed training and time to undertake a focused science project.
- Enrolment for PhD study is usually on a full-time basis. A PhD programme usually requires greater involvement in the laboratory environment with more emphasis on basic science.

3. *MD or PhD?* Long-term career plans are a major factor in deciding whether to undertake a higher degree and if so which. Regardless of whether a PhD does actually provide a better research training, this is the perception of grant-giving bodies and therefore a PhD is more appropriate for trainees considering a career in academic medicine and improves success in grant applications.

In contrast, if the aim is simply career advancement with plans to become an NHS consultant then an MD is more appropriate. However, undertaking an MD does not exclude the possibility of subsequently undertaking a career in academic medicine.

## Undertaking a successful research project

1. *Developing a research idea.*

- Discuss your general area of interest with your potential supervisor who should be able to provide guidance on which areas are potentially important research issues.
- With further reading you should be able to identify an idea for further discussion and development.
- Your potential supervisor may have a project already developed in your area of interest. Even though a project has already been developed this does not necessarily mean it would not be useful to take on the work as it will be possible to develop the project further, based on your own ideas and then subsequently based on your initial results.
- It is important to consider how risky the research project is with regard to how difficult it will be to get funding, obtain results and achieve publication.

2. **Expectations.** Junior doctors are used to structured timetables but in a research placement such structure is absent and the researcher is responsible for organization of his or her working time. The drafting and redrafting of protocols, grant applications, and ethical approvals give the impression of lack of productivity, which can be stressful initially.

3. **Realistic targets.** The time taken to undertake each stage within a research project will be grossly under-estimated. It is important not to be discouraged if the anticipated timetable for the project is not met.

4. **Patient recruitment and data collection.** It is essential not to rely on others to undertake your research project. They will not recruit subjects for your project and data will not collect itself. Staff under pressure to provide a service commitment will simply not prioritize your research project. If you must use other staff to assist in a project, their involvement must be kept as simple as possible and they should be engaged as much as possible by explaining why the project is being undertaken so that they feel they are part of a useful endeavour.

In summary, the fundamentals of good research are a good idea with a clear hypothesis, examined using a rigorous method, undertaken under the supervision of an experienced supervisor with adequate infrastructure and an enthusiastic and dedicated researcher.

## Further reading

Anderson M, Jankowski J. Higher research degrees: making the right choice. *British Medical Journal* 2001; **322:** S2–3.

Hull A, Guthrie M. Full-time research placement as a higher trainee. *British Medical Journal* 2000; **320:** S2–3.

Hüsler J, Wernecke KD. How to design trials/studies. In: Zbinden AM, Thomson D, (eds). *Conducting Research in Anaesthesia and Intensive Care Medicine.* Oxford: Butterworth Heinemann, 2001, pp. 97–138.

Pencheon D. Doing research. *British Medical Journal* 1999; **318:** S2–3.

Royal College of Physicians. *Guidelines for clinicians entering research* (1997) London: The Royal College of Physicians.

## Related topics of interest

Research process, p. 6; Laboratory research, p. 17; Audit, p. 188.

# RESEARCH PROCESS

*Somnath Chatterjee*

---

This topic outlines a systematic approach to a research project.

## Choosing a topic and a supervisor

You may have a question in mind, and choose a supervisor who is willing to help you, or you may choose a supervisor with a track record in research in an area of interest and select a topic offered. Discussion with colleagues will often provide useful information.

## Reviewing the literature

- The purpose of the review of literature is to gain insight into the current state of knowledge on the subject.
- Identifying material of interest has become easier with the wider availability of Index Medicus on CD-ROM and web-based search engines.
- Retrieving the articles or topics of interest and reading through them is time consuming so it is useful to set goals for the completion of this stage.
- Good note keeping during the review will significantly reduce the time needed to write a review of literature.

## Stating the hypothesis

A hypothesis is often a hunch that the researcher has about the existence of a relationship between variables. It defines the focus of the study. It may be possible to make minor modifications to the objectives as the study proceeds.

## Project outline

This helps to convey the study plan to your supervisor.

- It should consist of a working title, aims of the study and brief description of the questions to be answered and how you hope to answer them.
- A brief outline of the timetable at this stage helps to set goals for the study.
- Advice from a statistician will help to decide the tests that will be required to interpret the data. It will also give you an idea of the number of subjects that will be required to reach meaningful conclusions.

## Record keeping and note making

It is impossible to over-stress the importance of good record keeping and note making. To find information once is often tedious; to find it again when needed is virtually impossible. Familiarity with a card index system or software such as Excel™ or Access™ will prove invaluable later in the project. Software to manage your references (e.g. Reference Manager™) is a useful additional tool.

## Registering your research project

- It is a requirement of the Research Governance Framework of the Department of Health, that all projects are registered with the Department of Research and Development in your Trust.

- Following registration, the Department of Research and Development must review and approve your project on behalf of the Trust before it can be initiated.
- They may also provide assistance in writing up the protocol for submission to the Local Research Ethics Committee (LREC), helping one to avoid rejection for minor and often easily remediable mistakes.

## Research protocol

This is a detailed description of the planned project. It includes a title, the hypothesis, brief review of the literature, design of the trial, patient inclusion/exclusion criteria, measurements and details of the intended statistical analysis. The patient information sheet and consent form are also included. This document is submitted to the local research ethics committee (LREC) for approval.

## Ethical approval

All clinical research involving deviation from routine or accepted clinical practice will require approval from the LREC. This body is composed of doctors and nurses from various backgrounds and several lay people (see 'Research ethics committees', p. 55). It is vital to explain the present state of knowledge, purpose and methodology of the project and any risks involved, with great clarity. The patient information sheet and the consent form often delay ethical approval for lack of simplicity, clarity or honesty.

## Funding

Adequate funding is vital for successful completion of the project.

- It is important to take into account the time required to complete the project (salary of the researcher), laboratory tests involved, additional equipment or accessories, disposables, etc.
- The Department of Research and Development may help you to identify and apply for funding from other sources. Royal Colleges, speciality organizations, the British Medical Association and pharmaceutical companies will often part-fund projects. The Medical Research Council and Wellcome Trust mainly fund established research workers and expensive projects.

## Data collection

This is the process of gathering information to test the hypothesis.

- Being systematic and thorough during data collection will significantly improve the quality of the data and thereby improve the chances of reaching a meaningful conclusion.
- It is better to collect all possible data (within reasonable limits), than to be sorry at a later stage.
- If the data are being stored on a computer, always make adequate backups to insure against data loss. The computer should be registered with the Data Protection Commission.
- It is a good idea to store the paper version (either hand-written or printouts) in a safe place.
- Regular inspection and analysis of data for quality will help to identify problems early.

### Interpretation of data

Raw data mean nothing until they are analysed and presented systematically. Small projects do not often need detailed statistical analysis. Basic statistical knowledge and the ability to use statistical software is a great help. The Department of Research and Development should have specialists able to help.

### Writing the report

Report writing should not be a frantic activity at the end of the project.

- Disciplined record keeping and note making will greatly reduce the difficulties involved in writing up the report.
- Aim to establish the foundations of the report at the planning stage.
- Provide adequate time for writing up because this stage invariably involves multiple drafts before a satisfactory manuscript is completed.

### Presenting a paper

This often represents a highlight at the end of months of scientific endeavour.

- Deciding on the main message of the presentation, knowing the time allocated, having an idea about the audience, familiarity with presentation software (e.g. PowerPoint™), following basic rules while preparing the audio-visual aids and adequate practice form the foundation for a successful presentation.

### Writing a paper for publication

The results of the study are of no value unless they reach a relevant audience. Publication may also enhance your *curriculum vitae* and career prospects.

- It is vital to give the choice of journal a great deal of thought. The focus of the study will often govern the type of journal most likely to accept the article.
- Obtain and follow the instructions to authors with care.
- Decide on the authorship early in the project.
- It is unusual to have your first article accepted without modification. More often, you will be requested to make changes before it is accepted.
- Rejection may indicate a mistake in journal choice.

## Further reading

Department of Health. *Research Governance Framework*. London: Department of Health, 2001.
Medical Research Council. *MRC Guidelines for Good Clinical Practice in Clinical Trials*. London, Medical Research Council, 1998.
Medical Research Council. *Good Research Practice*. London, Medical Research Council, 2000.
O'Brien PMS, Pipkin FB. *Introduction to Research Methodology for Specialists and Trainees*. London, Royal College of Obstetricians and Gynaecologists, 1999.

## Related topics of interest

# RESEARCH IDEAS

*Tar-Ching Aw*

How does one start on research? What is required initially is a research question – and obviously this should be a question that has not already been answered. A search through the published literature in the medical and scientific databases will give an early indication of whether there are already many research papers dealing with that issue. Discussion with colleagues in the field will also help determine if the specific research question is worth pursuing.

## Avenues for research ideas

What is the source of a research question for a new researcher? There are several possible avenues.

*1. Clinical observation and practice.* In the course of clinical practice, a physician may make an observation about a clinical sign, technique or procedure or method of treatment, and this may lead to a question that can be answered by a research project. For example, if it is observed that a proportion of patients with alcoholic liver cirrhosis seem to present with Dupuytren's contracture, then one could well ask whether this is just a chance finding, or whether there is a definite link between the two conditions. If the association between the underlying medical condition and the clinical sign is confirmed, it could be a valuable sign in the diagnosis of alcoholic liver cirrhosis. This could form the basis of the research question.

*2. Trawling the literature.* When reading journal papers or articles in the medical literature, the author/s may pose a research question. The reader can adopt or modify that to formulate his/her own research question. It would be a useful part of the research process if the reader also has some ideas on the possible methods that can be used to answer the research question. At times, several articles on the same topic in the medical literature may all point to the same unanswered research questions. There may also be occasions when there appears to be conflicting information in the literature. A research study may come to a different conclusion from another study, and an individual beginning in research may wonder why this is so. The details of the study design or methodology used or interpretation may explain some of the contradictory findings. And it may even lead to a proposal for a better or different study to resolve some of the apparently conflicting information.

*3. Continuing professional development (CPD) activities.* Research ideas may emerge in the course of following CPD or continuing medical education (CME) activities. This includes attending presentations at scientific meetings or conferences, and discussions at seminars and workshops.

*4. Media attention.* Programmes on television and items in newspapers on health issues may form the basis of a research question. Media attention can reflect public interest in an issue. Some examples include the controversy over use of mobile phones and brain tumours, exposure to organophosphate pesticides in sheep dip and health effects, the Gulf War syndrome, ill-health in military personnel from exposure to spent uranium shells, etc. It is uncertain whether the alleged links between exposure and health effects are real, and research into the area may provide a clearer view. Concerns about an increase in spontaneous abortions and use of visual display terminals led to a number of research questions that formed the basis of large-scale epidemiological investigations showing the absence of a link.

**5. Audit findings.** Many organizations, including the National Health Service, have regular audits of their activities. Audit enables the assessment of progress in service delivery, facilitates implementation of remedial action and improvement of service provisions. Discussions at audit meetings and findings from audit processes may lead to the formulation of research questions. For example, auditing a Hepatitis B immunization programme can result in the question 'Should determination of antibody status be done before and after immunization, or is it sufficient just to check antibody levels after vaccination?' This question can form the basis of a research project.

**6. Funding agencies.** Organizations and agencies that fund research, e.g. the Medical Research Council, the Wellcome Foundation, and the Health and Safety Executive may publish a list of research topics for which funding is available. The topics indicate gaps in current knowledge and point to possibilities for research. A new researcher can use such lists to formulate research questions, prepare a research protocol and submit this for research funding. Such lists may also emerge following invitations from funding agencies for submission of research ideas for consideration. Publications and information from these agencies can be a ready source for research ideas.

**7. Self-generated research questions.** Occasionally, someone interested in research may initiate a research question just through cogitating about a particular medical or scientific topic. This may result because the individual has a specific interest in that topic. Or perhaps it is part of the inquisitive nature of potential successful researchers.

## Conclusion

There are many possibilities for posing research questions and finding research ideas. It is helpful for a new researcher not to be overwhelmed by a multitude of research questions. This tends to confuse and may make research appear to be an unmanageable activity. It is often best to limit the research questions to a few important issues. And each research question should be clear, concise and answerable.

## Further reading

Aw TC. Research methodology. *Occupational Medicine* 1997; **47**: 311–312.

Henig RM. *A monk and two peas: the story of Gregor Mendel and the discovery of genetics.* London: Weidenfeld and Nicolson, 2000.

Sackett DL, Haynes RB, Tugwell P. *Clinical epidemiology: a basic science for clinical medicine.* Boston: Little, Brown & Company, 1985.

## Related topics of interest

Medical research as part of post-graduate training, p. 1; Research process, p. 6.

# LITERATURE SEARCHING

*Lesley Allen*

Literature searching forms the backbone of any research project. Without preparing thoroughly, a researcher may find that someone else has already carried out the same or a similar piece of work. It is vital that the researcher sees what has already been published and what has not been studied in the field, sees how other studies were carried out and what problems were encountered.

This topic will assume a certain familiarity with the basic mechanics of searching and therefore this is written with the intention of giving hints and tips for a more effective and comprehensive search.

## What to search

*1. **MEDLINE.*** MEDLINE covers a wide range of subjects including medicine, nursing, dentistry, clinical science and veterinary science. It is a good place to start with regard to finding primary and current research. The database starts at 1966 and can be searched in date segments.

It is produced by the National Library of Medicine (NLM) and contains over 11 million journal citations and abstracts from approximately 4500 journals. All MEDLINE citations are assigned MeSH terms (Medical Subject Headings) and publication types from NLM's controlled vocabulary.

MEDLINE is available in a number of formats. It is commonly searched using either CD ROM or internet versions produced by commercial companies such as OVID. It is also available to users freely over the internet from a number of locations, including NLM in the form of PubMed. PubMed is slightly different from MEDLINE in that it will include for example citations preceding the date the journal was added to MEDLINE for indexing and also include some 'out of scope' citations from certain MEDLINE journals. Other organizations provide access to MEDLINE. A good place to look is www.omni.ac.uk/. OMNI (Organising Medical Networked Information) provides a table of MEDLINE services with information about registration, coverage and whether the service is free or not.

*2. **CINAHL.*** CINAHL (Cumulative Index of Nursing and Allied Health Literature) primarily covers literature of interest to nurses and other non-medical healthcare professionals. Its content is smaller than MEDLINE, indexing over 1200 journals, with about 70% of its index terms appearing in MEDLINE. These terms are supplemented by over 2000 other terms specifically designed to reflect nursing and allied health (see *Table 1*).

**Table 1.** Databases of MEDLINE and CINAHL

| Database | Since year | Number of references | Number of journals indexed | Number of index terms |
|---|---|---|---|---|
| MEDLINE | 1966 | 11 000 000 | 4500 | 19 000 |
| CINAHL | 1982 | 623 059 | 1296 | 11 094 |

## Evidence-based medicine

The Cochrane Library is a primary source for clinical effectiveness information. It is available freely on NELH (National Electronic Library for Health) to those using the NHSnet or registered with Athens, or by subscription to others.

- It contains four databases and provides evidence in the form of reviews and systematic reviews of the effectiveness of healthcare interventions/treatments. It is considered to be the gold standard in sources of evidence.
- In the first issue for 2002, there were 62 new Cochrane reviews and 55 reviews that had been substantially updated. There were also new protocols for a further 119 Cochrane reviews. As a result, the Cochrane Database of Systematic Reviews now contains the full text for nearly 1300 full reviews and more than 1000 protocols for reviews that are in preparation. 124 abstracts were added to the Database of Abstracts of Reviews of Effectiveness, during the last quarter, bringing its total to just short of 3300.
- The task facing the Cochrane Collaboration in reviewing healthcare research is seen in the growing size of CENTRAL (the Cochrane Controlled Trials Register). This contains bibliographic records for reports of studies that might be eligible for inclusion in Cochrane Reviews and is based mainly on the searching done around the world by members of the Cochrane Collaboration. It now contains more than a third of a million records.
- Just as Cochrane Reviews aim to bring together the most reliable evidence on the effects of health care, the reviews themselves aim to use the best evidence in the way they are undertaken. In recognition of this, the Cochrane Database of Methodology Reviews was added to The Cochrane Library in 2001. Information on individual studies or reports relating to the conduct of systematic reviews and other evaluations of health care are brought together in the Cochrane Methodology Register.

## The World Wide Web

The World Wide Web (WWW) is a useful and growing resource of information.

- If the address (URL) of the website you are interested in is known to you, you can go straight to it. Alternatively, you can search for the website or information you need using a search engine. Many websites will provide hypertext links to other useful webpages.
- There are a variety of search engines on the internet, e.g google, altavista. Be aware of the differences in each engine by experimenting and using the help on screen.
- There are also specific subject gateways that provide access to subject-specific web material. The benefit of using a gateway is that the websites on it have been pre-selected and therefore there is less chance of retrieving irrelevant material. Useful subject gateways include:
  http://omni.ac.uk – Organising Medical Networked Information
  http://sosig.ac.uk – Social Sciences Information Gateway
  http://www.medmatrix.org/index.asp – Medical Matrix gateway to clinical information
  http://medweb.emory.edu/ – MedWeb gateway to clinical information.

## Planning a search

The key to literature searching is preparation. The search question should be clearly defined. The more defined the question is, the more likely it is that relevant information will be retrieved.

*1. To define a search question.* The first stage in planning a search is to define the clinical question. The clinical question can be broken down into four parts, although certain parts may not be relevant in all cases.

(a) *The patient or population* – who is the question about?
(b) *The intervention or exposure* – what is being done or what is happening to the population?
(c) *Are there any comparisons?* – what could be done instead?
(d) *The outcome* – how does what is being done affect the population?

This can be remembered using the pneumonic PICO.

*2. Demonstration.* What follows is an example of how it works in practice:

(a) *The Question – PICO.* What is the incidence of Horner's Syndrome following central venous line insertion (see *Table 2(a)*)? This question has no comparison so this section can be left blank.
(b) *Key words or phrases.* This table can now be used to identify keywords, synonyms, spelling variations and alternative names or phrases (see *Table 2(b)*).
(c) *Combined subjects.* This structure is then used to plan the way subjects are combined (see *Table 2(c)*).

## Methods of searching bibliographic databases

Bibliographic databases are made up of records. Each record contains a number of fields such as author, title, publication year, keywords, etc. Each of these fields is searchable and searches can be restricted to particular fields or can be freetext. It is

**Table 2(a).** Planning a search

| Patient or problem | Intervention | Comparison | Outcome |
|---|---|---|---|
| Horner's syndrome | Central venous line insertion | | Incidence |

**Table 2(b).** Planning a search

| Patient or problem | Intervention | Comparison | Outcome |
|---|---|---|---|
| Horner's syndrome | Central venous line insertion | | Incidence |
| Horner syndrome MeSH HEADING | Central venous line Central venous line catheterisation/ catheterization Cannulation MeSH HEADING | | |

**Table 2(c).** Planning a search

| Patient or problem | | Intervention | Comparison | | Outcome |
|---|---|---|---|---|---|
| Horner's syndrome | and | Central venous line insertion | | and | Incidence |
| or | | | | | |
| Horner syndrome | and | Central venous line | | and | |
| or | | | | | |
| MeSH heading | and | Central venous line catheterisation/ catheterization | | and | |
| or | | | | | |
| | and | Cannulation | | and | |
| or | | | | | |
| | and | MeSH heading | | and | |

also possible to search specific things in specific fields at the same time. Different databases may also have different ways of expressing the author's name, etc. It is worth having a look at the help available before beginning a search if you are unclear.

**1.  Controlled vocabulary.** The controlled vocabulary of MEDLINE is known as MeSH (Medical Subject Headings). Those responsible for indexing the records on MEDLINE select terms from this list to reflect the subject content of the articles indexed. Each article is given a number of these MeSH headings to reflect its content. Therefore articles on similar subjects will be indexed under the same terms, which makes it easier to find all relevant information. For example, all papers on heart attacks have been indexed under myocardial infarction. Many MEDLINE search interfaces are designed so that they translate words entered into MeSH terms automatically.

**2.  Free text.** It is also possible, and advisable, to search using free text. By searching this way it is possible to search more than just the index terms, but any part of the reference including title and abstract. This is particularly useful if what you are looking for is a new concept. Also it is useful as it will enable you to carry out a comprehensive search, picking up those anomalies that have crept into the system. However, searching in this way will only retrieve records containing the exact phrase you have entered. For example, *woman* will not retrieve *women* or *female*.

**3.  Subheadings.** Several common concepts such as adverse effects, complications, diagnosis and so on are covered by what are known as subheadings. These are appended to the MeSH term. These are quite useful for general references about specific subjects, for example drug treatment in asthma.

**4.  Limiting.** If your search is not very specific it may yield a large number of references. It is possible to refine the search further. The selection of limits includes the language of the paper, publication year, age groups, human or animal subjects and publication types to name just a few. Using the limits can be useful in reducing the number of references in a set if it is unmanageable. However, limiting to a particular language could exclude potentially important research.

5. **Methodological filters.** Methodological filters, sometimes referred to as search filters, are another way of limiting searches. Many are based on expert searches originally developed by McMaster University in Canada. They are designed in such a way that they are able to identify sound clinical studies of the aetiology, prognosis, diagnosis, prevention or treatment of disorders. In addition, there are also filters to identify systematic reviews and clinical trials. Methodological filters are never used alone, but in combination with a subject search. The following web address provides links to filters: http://www.shef.ac.uk/~scharr/ir/filter.html

6. **Boolean operators.** Boolean operators are used to combine parts of the search together in various ways. The three operators are: AND, OR, NOT. Each of these operators will have a different effect on the outcome of the search. AND – narrows the search to find records containing both (or all) of the search terms combined, e.g. coronary disease AND exercise will retrieve references where both terms are present. OR – broadens the search by retrieving all or any of the search terms combined, e.g. coronary disease OR exercise will retrieve references where either term is present. NOT – excludes one or more of the search terms, e.g. (coronary disease AND exercise) NOT men will retrieve references on exercise in coronary heart disease, but not in men. The NOT operator can be useful for refining the results of a search but should always be used with caution as it is possible to exclude some potentially relevant references.

7. **Other hints and tips.** These hints are particularly relevant to enhancing the free-text search.

- Truncation – (usually $ or *) is a useful way of retrieving all words beginning with a particular string. For example: imag$3.tw. for words like image, images, imagine but not imagination.
- Nesting ( ) operator, e.g. (pregnancy and childbirth).ti. for both pregnancy and childbirth in the title.
- Adjacency (adj) operator – will look for the exact phrase you type in such as diverticular adj absess.
- Synonyms, e.g. use family practice as well as general practice.
- Variant spelling, e.g. color and colour.
- When search skills are developed it is possible to type search statements directly into the command line. In doing this it is possible to short cut some of the more drawn out methods of searching, for example: stroke.ti. not bmj.so. will look for references about stroke, but not those that appeared in the British Medical Journal (BMJ).
- Command line searching is a more advanced skill and should be used carefully until the mechanisms are understood fully.
- Checking the help for the database being used should provide help on the command line syntax used.

## Improving your search skills

The best way of improving search skills is to practice. Most of the versions of Medline available have online help available to assist you when you are searching. Also your local health service librarian will be able to offer help and guidance in search skills.

## Further reading

Alper J. Assembling the world's biggest library on your desktop. *Science* 1998; **281:** 1784–1786.

Greenhalgh T. *How to read a paper. The basics of evidence based medicine.* 2nd ed. BMJ Publishing Group, 2001.

## Related topic of interest

Writing up: case reports, publications and thesis, p. 176; Systematic reviews and meta-analysis, p. 167; Research ideas, p. 8.

# LABORATORY RESEARCH

*Daqing Ma*

Laboratory research differs from other kinds of research in that the experimental conditions can be well controlled and hence a specific point can be investigated in detail. This is a complex topic and only the fundamental issues will be discussed here.

## Process of laboratory research

A completed piece of laboratory research, like all other kinds of research, involves *four stages*:

- researching the background knowledge;
- designing the study protocol and doing the work;
- analysing and presenting the data;
- publishing the work.

*1. Background knowledge.* This is like the foundations of a building. Before working on any project, investigators should search widely for, and read, the publications in the specific field to find out:

- what has been done;
- what has not been done;
- is there any established protocol and experimental model available.

One must have such general information in the particular field because it will help not only in setting up a topic to study but also in designing the experimental protocol.

*2. Hypothesis.* A hypothesis is the key to the work to be undertaken. It may not only reflect the quality of the work, but also indicate the investigators' knowledge of the field. Laboratory work should have a clear hypothesis simply because any influencing factors on the results can be eliminated and specific points can be properly investigated. However, this does not imply that the hypothesis is always correct or that positive results will always be obtained.

*3. Experimental protocol.* This should be designed to be both feasible and logical. Full details should be included of all apparatus and materials which will be used and any published methods cited. If animals are involved, the protocol must be approved by the relevant animal welfare authority. In the United Kingdom, this will involve adherence to the Animals (Scientific Procedures) Act, 1986. If the study involves humans, approval of the protocol by the local research ethics committee is needed. In order to reduce systematic error, allocation to experimental groups should be done randomly.

*4. Laboratory notes and discussion.* In the process of writing the laboratory notes, there is a need to follow through the experimental process mentally with great care so that potential errors may be picked up at an early stage. Any unclear points may be clarified by the process of careful writing. Oral reports of preliminary results or new ideas within the group, team, or department are also very helpful because criticisms raised at this stage are particularly useful. The preliminary results should be also submitted to an appropriate learned society because the feedback and questions arising from other people working in the same field are helpful in completing a project.

**5. Manuscript.** A publishable manuscript should be precise, succinct, clear and readable. It is quite different from a degree thesis or a general report. The Discussion section of the manuscript should not be too long. If it is written like a review, it will not be welcomed by reviewers or editors or indeed by well-informed readers.

(a) *Authorship.* Every author should contribute adequate work to the paper and also accept responsibility to the public for their contribution. Anyone giving technical assistance should be included in the acknowledgements.

(b) *Structure.* Each journal has its own structural format for articles. Commonly used formats are:
- *Medical paper.* Introduction, Methods or Materials and Methods, Results and Discussion, Summary or Abstract (which may appear first).
- *Scientific survey.* Introduction, Geographical and Historical Context, Fieldwork, Analysis of Results, Discussion and Conclusion.
- *Theoretical paper.* Introduction, Theoretical Analysis, Application and Conclusions.
- *New Methods.* Introduction, Description of Procedure, Tests of New Method, Discussion.

**6. Submission of manuscript.** In general, it is acceptable for similar material to be published as an abstract and as a formal paper, but multiple publication of the same data is unacceptable. Where the manuscript should be submitted depends on the quality of the work and the particular scientific field. It should ideally be published where other relevant researchers will read it – not necessarily in a prestigious general journal.

## Further Reading

Laurence N, Perks C, Farndon JR. Laboratory-based research. *British Medical Journal*, Career Focus 2001; **323**: 2.

## Related topics of interest

Research process, p. 6; Writing up: case report, publications and thesis, p. 176.

# RESEARCH INVOLVING ANIMALS

*YinHua Zhang*

Animals are pivotal in biomedical research. As the demand for animals in scientific research increases and the results permeate into everyday life, it is important to understand the guidelines before proceeding to experiments with animals. The concept of preventing cruelty to animals in the laboratory was introduced in the 19th century. Following decades of modification, the Animal (Scientific Procedures) Act 1986 was passed to define the duties and responsibilities of all those involved in animal research.

## Animals

A licence is required under the 1986 Act for any experiment involving a 'regulated procedure' on 'protected animals'.

*1. Regulated procedures* are those which cause pain, suffering, distress or lasting harm.

*2. Protected animals* are defined as all living vertebrate animals except man. They are in two groups:

- Mammals, birds and reptiles, from halfway through the gestation or incubation period.
- Fish, amphibians and the cephalopod mollusc, *Octopus vulgaris*, from the time that they become capable of independent feeding.

Under the Act, an animal is regarded as alive until the cessation of circulation or destruction of its brain: procedures carried out on decerebrate animals are therefore subject to the controls.

## Types of licence

Two kinds of licence are required for all scientific work controlled under the Act, a personal licence and a project licence, both of which are granted by the Home Office on the advice of their local inspector.

*1. Project licence.* This is required when a programme of work uses live animals for a purpose permitted by the Act. It will be granted where the Home Office Inspector considers that the use of live animals is appropriate for the scientific research in question. The applicant for a project licence must be credible and must undertake overall responsibility for the scientific direction and control of the work. The project licence holder will generally be the senior personal holder engaged on the project. Regulated procedures on living animals may not be performed on the authority of a project licence alone. There must also be a personal licence.

*2. Personal licence.* A personal licence is the Home Secretary's endorsement of the holder's competence and suitability to carry out specified procedures on specified animals. A personal licence is required for anyone who is using a regulated procedure. The procedure must be part of a programme of work authorized by a project licence. No work may be done unless the procedure, the animals used, and the place where the work is done are specifically authorized in both the personal and project licences. Applicants must be at least 18 years of age and are required to provide details of their qualifications, training and experience. Once issued, the personal licence will be in force continuously until revoked, but the Home Secretary reviews each licence at intervals not exceeding 5 years.

The personal licensee is personally responsible for ensuring:

(a) that all his or her animals are clearly identifiable;
(b) that steps are taken to reduce any suffering to a minimum consistent with the scientific procedure;
(c) that they comply with the termination conditions, so that any animal in severe pain or severe distress which cannot be alleviated must be killed at once;
(d) that the procedure is authorized by a project licence and is being carried out in a designated place;
(e) that records are kept;
(f) that the animal cages are labelled.

## Designation of premises

All places where regulated scientific procedures are performed must be designated by a certificate issued by the Home Secretary, unless otherwise authorized in the project and personal licences. In addition, establishments which breed certain types of animals for use in scientific procedures must be designated. The Certificate of Designation is issued to the person who represents the governing authority of the establishment and who is ultimately responsible to the Home Office for ensuring that the conditions of the certificate are observed.

## Euthanasia and 'Schedule 1'

The 1986 Act requires the humane killing of experimental animals, which is called Schedule 1.

*1. The techniques.* These are:

- confirmation of permanent cessation of the circulation;
- destruction of the brain;
- dislocation of the neck;
- exsanguination;
- confirmation of the onset of *rigor mortis*;
- instantaneous destruction of the body in a macerator.

If the technique of killing is not listed in Schedule 1, then it will need to be specifically authorized under the Act.

*2. Specific authorization.* Even if the personal licensee uses Schedule 1, if any manipulation or experimental procedure is undergone, it should be considered as 'a regulated procedure' that requires specific authorization. The actual killing of the animal using Schedule 1 does not necessarily require a personal licence. However, it should be carried out by a competent person and in a designated place. The university (or responsible person in any other designated place) is responsible for ensuring this.

*3. Re-use of animals.* Caution should be exercised when considering the re-use of animals after one procedure is finished with the intention of proceeding to another because it needs to be specifically authorized by the Home Office. Generally, if an animal undergoes a procedure that requires anaesthesia, re-use will not normally be permitted.

## Special aspects of conducting medical research using animals

*1. Selection of the animal model.* A successful animal research project depends upon the match of the research question to the appropriate animal model. The aim of using an animal model is to extrapolate experimental findings to humans. Researchers usually use easily accessible, relatively inexpensive species. However, the validity of the extrapolation depends on the similarities of the chosen species to humans as well as the target organ system. For example, an applicable model for human brain protection is a non-human primate such as a monkey or chimpanzee. The coronary circulation of the dog has a rich collateral circulation, and canine studies therefore may not be directly applicable to humans. In fact, the porcine coronary circulation more closely resembles that of humans.

*2. The ethical aspects.* The experimenter should be conversant with the techniques of handling, restraint and injection of animals. Efforts should be made to minimize the distress that can be caused to animals in an effort to obtain good scientific results. The 1986 Act requires that experimenters should be capable of recognizing pain and distress in their animals. Procedures must, therefore, be categorized into mild, moderate and substantial.

*3. Laboratory species.* It is important for research workers to have a basic knowledge of the biology of the laboratory species that they use in their work. Animals should be housed appropriately within a suitable environment, having regard to temperature, humidity, ventilation, lighting and noise.

*4. 'Alternatives'.* In animal experimentation, the term 'alternatives' has a special meaning. The concept embraces the three Rs:

(a) *Reduction* – reducing the number of animals required;
(b) *Refinement* – diminishing the amount of pain or distress;
(c) *Replacement* – considering whether it is possible to replace the need for animal experimentation.

*5. Safety.*

(a) *Injury.* The hazards of working with laboratory animals include the risk of physical injury caused by animals. In order to avoid unexpected injury it is vital for the animal handler to appreciate the normal behaviour and possible defensive tactics of the species to be used. First-aid facilities and a person trained in first-aid should be available in all places handling animals.
(b) *Diseases.* Like human beings, animals are susceptible to clinical diseases. These may be infectious (viral, bacterial, protozoal and metazoan parasites) or may be a consequence of toxic insults, physical injury, genetic malformations, neoplasia, etc. Although some infectious diseases are species specific, some are transmissible to another species, including humans. More importantly, animals are also susceptible to sub-clinical and chronic diseases. Research workers should therefore have a basic knowledge of the diseases to which their experimental animals are susceptible. The law requires that the health conditions be monitored routinely (Health Screen) in all places which house animals.

(c) *Allergy.* Allergy to laboratory animals (ALA) is a relatively common disorder which some individuals develop in the course of their work. The use of special hygiene procedures (e.g. ventilated cages, ceiling-to-floor air flow, protective clothing (gloves, gown, mask), special care in handling excreta etc.) help prevent ALA.

**6. *Security.*** Whilst every effort is made to avoid cruelty to animals during scientific procedures, all animal users need to be aware that there is an increasing public awareness of, and hostility to, the use of animals in medical and scientific research. The following guidelines are highly recommended to maximize security:

- Do not broadcast your activities;
- Do not leave sensitive documents lying around for all to read;
- Do not allow access to your facilities by unknown persons;
- Make full use of the security measures provided by the institution;
- Inform the police or the institutional security service if you receive unexpected items by post or receive strange or abusive phone calls.

## Further Reading

*Home Office Code of Practice for the Housing and Care of Animals Used in Scientific Procedures.* House of Commons Paper 107, HMSO, 1989, London.
*Home Office Guidance on the Operation of the Animals (Scientific Procedures).* House of Commons Paper 182. HMSO: London, 1990.
Wolfensohn S, Lloyd M. *Handbook of Laboratory Animal Management and Welfare.* Oxford: Oxford University Press, 1994.

## Related topic of interest

Laboratory research, p. 17.

# VOLUNTEER STUDIES

*Taj Dhallu*

Clinical research needs to be carried out to determine if a proposed new treatment is going to benefit patients. Clinical research can be observational or experimental. Observational research may involve measurement such as height, blood pressure or survival time, while experimental research involves the application of different treatments to different groups of subjects. Experimental clinical research is organized in the form of clinical trials.

## Clinical trials

Experimental research is carried out on humans only after the safety of the treatment has been assessed in animals. Clinical trials on humans are designed and organized into four phases, phase I, II, III and IV.

- Phase I of the clinical trial usually involves healthy volunteers who are subjected to the proposed treatment. The objective of a phase I trial is to gather data on the safety, acceptability, side-effect profile, suitable dose, and the pharmacokinetic and pharmacodynamic properties of the new drug in man.
- In phase II, III and IV trials, patients with a specific target disease are recruited as subjects.
- The difference between the phases is that an increasing number of patients are involved.

## Ethics and human volunteers

1. **Coercion.** It is absolutely essential that individuals are not persuaded to volunteer for clinical trials.

- Clinical trials are often carried out in hospitals where there are many medical students and laboratory technicians willing to volunteer as subjects for these trials.
- It is extremely important to appreciate that such people may feel under pressure to volunteer because of a concern for their future career prospects. A similar situation arises in prisons or the armed services.

2. **Consent.** Volunteers must understand the nature, purpose and risks of a clinical trial.

- It is the responsibility of the investigator to explain in plain language that the subject may withdraw from the trial at any time without giving reasons and without fear of sanctions. Patients may be afraid to withdraw from a clinical trial because they feel they must keep on good terms with their physician to secure continuing treatment.
- An information sheet should be given to all research subjects, preferably at least one day before the study.
- Once the investigator is sure that the volunteer understands the clinical trial and the responsibilities of the volunteer, signed written consent should be obtained.

3. **Financial inducements.** Although some individuals volunteer for altruistic motives, many may do so because of financial rewards.

- The size of any payment should not be enough to act as an inducement but should cover such things as loss of earnings, inconvenience, travel expenses and a small amount for any discomfort.
- A record of all payments should be kept.

4. **Health of volunteers.** The investigator is responsible for ensuring that the subjects are fit for the demands of the study, especially in studies that involve a treatment.

- A thorough history and examination should be carried out.
- Permission to contact the General Practitioner should be sought to obtain further information on the health status of the individual and to alert the General Practitioner to the fact that the subject has volunteered for the study. Any inappropriate volunteering may then be detected.
- For in-patients, the permission of the consultant under whose care the patient has been admitted should be obtained.

5. **Female volunteers.** The investigators must bear in mind that a woman may be, or become, pregnant during the study; this has important implications for both the woman and the fetus.

- Women of child-bearing age are usually excluded from phase I, and sometimes phase II trials.
- The effect of the proposed treatment on breast-feeding must be understood.

6. **Potentially harmful treatments.**

- Therapeutic agents such as anti-cancer or immunosuppressive drugs may have harmful side effects. It is ethically unacceptable to subject healthy volunteers to these drugs. Patients with target diseases for such drugs are recruited for these studies.
- The inherent risks of the drug or treatment should be assessed against their potential benefits.

7. **Indemnity.** A fundamental principle of medical research is that subjects should not be exposed to danger. However, all treatments have known and unknown side effects. The results of animal experiments may not necessarily apply to human beings.

(a) *Individual researchers.* Because of this theoretical risk of harm, it is essential for both the investigator and the subjects to be legally protected.
(b) *Drug companies.* Pharmaceutical companies will indemnify the subjects against any injury resulting from the treatment unless it can be shown to be due to negligence on the part of the investigator.
(c) *The NHS Trust.* In the National Health Service, provided that the Local Research Ethics Committee has approved the study, the Trust will accept liability for damages caused by negligence. It is essential to ensure that these arrangements are in place.

## Conduct of a volunteer study

1. **Recruitment of human volunteers.** There are many reasons why individuals may volunteer to participate in a clinical trial and these range from an altruistic

desire to help medical science or to assist an individual doctor, right through to financial inducements or psychological motivation.

- Some individuals may volunteer because they suffer from a terminal illness such as cancer for which the new treatment may be a cure.
- Whatever the reason, there are ethical considerations and also statistical bias implications for the analysis of the data.

**2. *Place of investigation.*** The administration of any treatment, or experimental procedure such as blood sampling, should take place in an environment where there are adequate facilities for resuscitation including intubation, oxygenation and defibrillation.

**3. *Statistical implications.***

(a) *Bias from self-selection – 'volunteer bias'.*
- If the results of a clinical trial are to be applicable to the general population, everyone from that population should have an equal chance of being chosen to be a subject in the study. This implies random selection, but volunteers, by definition, are not chosen at random but self-selection.
- They tend to be better educated, healthier and have better hygiene than non-volunteers: this self-selection will cause volunteer bias.

(b) *Bias from demographic distribution.*
- Phase I studies are often restricted to males between the ages of 18 and 35 years who are not taking any medication and do not abuse alcohol. Young and healthy subjects are initially selected in the belief that they are more likely to tolerate any unforeseen side effects. Females are avoided because of the fear of damage to the fetus if the woman becomes pregnant.
- The limited age group and avoidance of women means that any data obtained may not be applicable to a different population. Older individuals may be on medication that may interact with the proposed treatment. Older patients also have less physiological reserve, particularly renal function, which may delay clearance of drugs.

(c) *Bias from motivation.*
- Volunteers may want to please the physician, and thus may exhibit symptoms of the success of the treatment. However, financial inducements may result in the recruitment of poorer and less-healthy individuals.

Because of these various biases, volunteer studies are restricted to Phase I of a clinical trial. In phase II or III trials the extent of bias should become clearer.

## Further Reading

Bland M. *An introduction to medical statistics*, 2nd edn. Oxford: Oxford University Press, 1995.
Weiskopf RB. How to perform volunteer studies. In: Zbinden AM, Thomson D (eds). *Conducting Research in Anaesthesia and Intensive Care Medicine*. Oxford: Butterworth-Heinemann, 2001, pp. 499–514.

## Related topics of interest

Research ethics committees, p. 55; Research process, p. 6; Research design, p. 31.

# QUALITATIVE RESEARCH

*Sukhbinder Singh*

Qualitative research has traditionally been the domain of social sciences such as anthropology and sociology. However, in recent years this type of research has become established as an important tool in medical and nursing health research. Many high-quality qualitative research studies are appearing in mainstream medical journals. Despite this, doctors and other health care professionals, who have traditionally been taught and practised quantitative research, are unfamiliar with qualitative research.

## What is qualitative research?

*1. Definition.* Qualitative research may be defined as the type of research that seeks an understanding and meaning of human thoughts, experiences, events, cultures and phenomena.

*2. Qualitative research process.* Unlike quantitative research there is no theory to be examined in a controlled experimental setting.

- In qualitative research the initial questions are often vague and broad.
- Data are collected by a variety of methods, the aim being to produce detailed and rich descriptions of various phenomena.
- The documentation of data is often in the form of words and pictures, which are then analysed and interpreted inductively to develop explanatory theories and concepts of the phenomena under study. These theories can then be tested deductively by quantitative research.

*3. An example.* An example would be a study looking at patient compliance with medication.

- A quantitative study may examine how many patients fail to comply and how frequently each patient fails to comply with his treatment.
- However, a qualitative study might examine what the patients' perception of compliance is and why they fail to comply.
- Of course, both approaches can be combined in a single study.

## Features of qualitative research

There are a number of distinctive features related to qualitative research. These include the following:

*1. Naturalistic.* Qualitative research is often termed naturalistic because the subjects are studied in their own natural environments. The data are obtained by observing and speaking to individuals in their surroundings. This is one of its strengths as the findings will be valid for the group studied, although they may not be generalizable to a wider population.

*2. Subject's perspective.* There is an emphasis on determining the meaning of phenomena, events and situations from the subject's perspective. To achieve this, the researchers have to suspend their own preconceptions and immerse themselves in the world of the subject.

3. **Evolution.** Studies evolve in their design as data are gathered and analysed. Usually, little information is available at the beginning of the study but, as more becomes known about the subject matter during the study, this knowledge is used to guide subsequent strategies including decisions about which data collection methods to use, what questions to ask and who to ask.

4. **Researcher.** The researcher is usually the main research instrument. This imposes significant responsibility on researchers who need to develop a friendly rapport with their subjects, show empathy and gain the trust of their subjects to facilitate an accurate, honest and frank disclosure.

5. **Sampling.** This should ensure that the whole spectrum of opinions, both typical and deviant, within a population is represented. Sampling is purposely designed to select those subjects who will reflect the widest diversity within a particular group. The sample size is usually small, consisting of between four and 40 subjects, who are studied in great detail.

6. **Thick description.** This term refers to in-depth and detailed descriptions of the issues being studied as opposed to a superficial commentary. The description includes rich details of the research setting, the context of the study, the individuals and what they say, their actions and relationships with others. This description may include photographs and actual quotations from the participants.

## Qualitative research methods

A number of methods are utilized in qualitative research which all share the features outlined above.

1. **Ethnography.** This attempts to describe and interpret certain aspects of culture such as behaviour, speech and beliefs. The culture under study may be broadly based such as that of a religious group, or be focused on a subculture such as a group of general practitioners in an inner-city practice. This type of study involves long periods of fieldwork, including interviewing many participants, which is then followed by detailed textual description so that the culture may be communicated to others.

2. **Phenomenology.** This originates from philosophy. It is a research approach that seeks to understand the life experiences of people and the meanings and interpretations people attach to those experiences or phenomena. Understanding the essence of this lived experience is achieved by in-depth conversations, usually with a small number of participants. Experiences that may be studied include birth, bereavement, stress, depression, diagnosis of a malignancy or quality of life with a chronic illness.

3. **Grounded theory.** This is used to systematically generate explanations or theories about human behaviour. The development of theory is 'grounded' in the dataset, rather than from *a priori* assumptions or other pre-existing theories. The data are collected (using interviews, observations and documents), analysed and compared simultaneously to develop hypotheses. Further sampling and data collection are used to verify the emerging hypotheses. These are then integrated to develop a theory that explains the phenomena under study. The theory is then subsequently tested.

## Data collection methods

Numerous data collection methods are utilized in qualitative research.

*1. **Observation**.* This relies on the researcher observing groups of people undergoing activities within their own environments, such as a group of nurses working in an Accident and Emergency department.

- It is used to document the behaviour, interactions and conversations of people in a systematic and detailed manner.
- The observation may be overt with the researcher simply watching the group in an unobtrusive manner. Observers may become participants in the group. This reduces the potential influence of the observer on the group and may allow more representative data to be obtained.
- Data collection is usually in the form of field notes that are taken simultaneously as the group is being observed or later if note-taking during observation is impractical or undesirable.

*2. **Interviews**.* These are the commonest form of data collection. The aim is to elicit information from the respondent's own perspective by asking clear, open-ended and neutral questions. It is important not to bias the interview by imposing one's own theories or assumptions onto the respondent. Interviews have been classified as:

(a) *Unstructured interviews.* Unstructured and in-depth – where only one or two issues are explored in great detail and where there may be little control of the interview by the researcher.
(b) *Semi-structured interviews.* Semi-structured – in which interviews are more focused, with a number of issues being explored and with greater control and direction of the interview by the interviewer.
(c) *Structured interviews.* Structured interviews – which are similar to written questionnaires and are infrequently used.

*3. **Focus groups**.* These are a form of interview that involves several participants interacting with each other to explore various issues.

- Group interaction may stimulate the development of thoughts and ideas that may not otherwise emerge in one-to-one interviews.
- The researcher facilitates discussion and prevents any individual from dominating the group.
- Widely used in marketing and advertising, this method is also used to assess various health-related topics such as the experience of certain illnesses, attitudes of health professionals and appraisal of health services.

*4. **Documents**.* Documents can be an important source of information, especially when the above data collection methods are not possible.

- Useful documents may include diaries, biographies, case notes and audio-visual records.
- They are analysed in the same way as the written records of observational fieldwork and transcripts of interviews.

## Analysing qualitative research

Transcriptions of interviews and focus groups, field notes from observational research and notes from other documents result in large amounts of textual data that require systematic and rigorous analysis.

- The purpose of analysis in qualitative research is to generate explanations or theories that explain the phenomena under study.
- Data collection and analysis usually take place simultaneously. This allows provisional hypotheses to develop and subsequently modify further data collection so that the emerging hypotheses may be examined in greater depth.
- For analysis to take place, complete familiarity with the data is important. This is achieved by studying the textual data repeatedly.
- As comprehension is achieved, categories and themes that explain the phenomena emerge from the data. These are coded and further categories identified.
- Software programmes may facilitate the coding of data.
- Data collection continues until no further categories emerge. Many categories may emerge from the data and these are refined together to develop key explanatory theories.
- The analysis may be conducted by more than one individual to improve reliability.

## Validity of qualitative research

Ensuring that the findings are valid is important. Errors can be introduced in a number of ways including observer bias and the Hawthorne effect (where the presence of the researcher affects the behaviour of the subjects). A number of strategies have been devised to improve the validity of qualitative research.

1. *Researcher biases.* Researchers should be aware of their biases and outline them in their written reports.

2. *Prolonged engagement.* This allows for in-depth understanding and reduces the impact of the researcher on the behaviour of the subjects.

3. *Negative cases.* Cases that fail to conform to the explanations being developed should be scrutinized to refine and improve the explanatory theories that are being generated.

4. *Triangulation.* This is the process of using different data collection techniques (such as interviews and observational fieldwork) to study the same phenomena. Consistency of findings with different data collection methods improves the credibility of the research.

5. *Respondent validation.* If subjects (respondents) check the research findings and agree with the observations and the explanations of the phenomena, the value of the research is enhanced.

## Further Reading

Denzin NK, Lincoln YS. *Handbook of Qualitative Research.* London: Sage, 1994.
Pope C, Mays N. *Qualitative Research in Health Care.* 2nd Edn. London: BMJ Publishing Group, 2000.

## Related topics of interest

Data collection, p. 64; Research process, p. 6.

# RESEARCH DESIGN

*Craig Jackson, John E. Smith*

In contrast to laboratory or animal research, clinical studies use patients or volunteers in an attempt to address questions of direct clinical significance. The aim of this topic is to present principles and guidelines on how to design clinical research.

## Types of clinical research

Clinical research may be broadly classified into experimental studies or observational studies. These may be further subdivided into longitudinal or cross-sectional and prospective or retrospective designs (*Figure 1*).

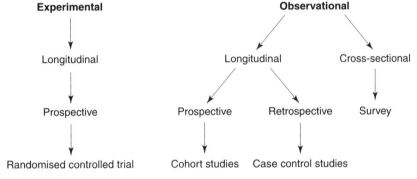

Figure 1. Types of clinical research.

*1. Experimental studies.* In experimental studies the investigator makes an intervention, for example gives a drug, then studies the effects of the intervention.

(a) *Features of experimental studies.*
- Particularly common forms of experimental trial are those involving comparisons or associations between two or more groups of patients.
- They are always longitudinal – they study changes in the subjects in response to the intervention over a period of time.
- They are always prospective – data are collected from the start of the study onwards.

(b) *Terminology.*
- Experimental studies are referred to as 'experimental trials', or 'clinical trials' or just 'trials'.
- Because they are typically randomized and controlled, they may also be referred to as 'randomized controlled trials'.
- They may also be blinded, although in some circumstances this may not be possible.

*2. Observational studies.* In observational studies the investigator observes, describes, analyses and interprets an existing or pre-existing situation but does nothing to influence events.

They may be longitudinal or cross-sectional.

(a) *Longitudinal observational studies.* Longitudinal studies may be divided into case–control studies and cohort studies.
- Case–control studies are retrospective, moving backwards in time from effect to cause (from disease to exposure).
- Cohort studies are prospective, moving forwards in time from cause to effect (from exposure to disease).

(b) *Cross-sectional observational studies.*
- Cross-sectional studies are surveys which examine subjects at just one point of time.
- They are often based on a random sample of a particular population, for example, patients presenting with a specific disease, medical students or smokers, etc.

## Experimental studies

*1. Purpose.* The purpose of an experimental trial is to evaluate the effectiveness of an intervention or therapy. The different interventions are applied to similar groups of individuals, who should reflect the population concerned. The differences in observed outcomes should therefore be a direct consequence of the relative efficacy of the interventions tested. Hence, the best evidence of cause and effect may be derived from this type of study.

*2. Types of experimental studies.* Experimental trials may study differences between subjects or within subjects.

(a) *Between subjects (independent data).*
- In parallel studies, each group of patients receives a different treatment or intervention concurrently.

(b) *Within subjects (paired data).*
- Within-subject designs have the important advantage that the subject acts as his or her own control and therefore between-subject variability is removed.
- In paired studies, measurements on each patient are taken more than once, usually in different circumstances, e.g. before and after treatment.
- In cross-over studies, each patient receives each treatment in sequence, with a 'washout' period between the two (or more) treatments. It is important that the order of the treatments is randomized.
- A matched-pairs design is a parallel study in which each subject in one arm is matched with a subject in the other arm for all known prognostic factors. These two groups are thus closely interrelated and therefore the data may be treated as paired.

## Principles of the design of experimental trials

This section discusses the established principles and methods upon which experimental trials are based.

*1. Avoiding bias.* The validity of the results of both experimental and observational studies depends on the extent to which investigators have been able to avoid all possible sources of bias.

(a) *Bias.*

- Bias is a systematic distortion of a result due to a factor not allowed for in the design of the study. For example, bias would occur if, when testing two different treatments, the two groups were given tablets that looked different; or if one group was given a tablet and the control group was not given a tablet. The two groups of patients are managed differently and it is possible that these differences might influence the trial results.

- A fundamental flaw in design might confound a trial, invalidating the results. For example, if the investigator, when studying the incidence of upper respiratory tract infections (URTI) in doctors and ancillary staff in a hospital, failed to take into account their smoking histories. It is likely that there would be a significant difference in this regard between the two groups. Therefore, it becomes impossible to distinguish the effects of occupation from the effects of smoking on the incidence of URTI.

(b) *Methods.*

- The control group, randomization and blinding are the classical techniques that have evolved to minimize bias in experimental trials.

## 2. Control group.

(a) *Importance.*

- When testing the effectiveness of a new treatment or procedure in medicine, it is essential to have a concurrent comparison, a control group, to whom the experimental treatment is not given. Without a control group it is impossible to make an objective evaluation of the effect (if any) of a treatment.

- There are many reasons why bias can occur in an uncontrolled or open study. Any increase in well-being or relief of symptoms experienced by the subjects cannot be safely ascribed to the treatment they have been given since the simple knowledge that they are receiving a treatment may alone have beneficial effects, even if the treatment is completely inactive (the placebo effect). The patients' responses may also be greatly influenced by the investigator's enthusiasm, optimism or (unconscious) reassurance, etc. Since the investigator knows exactly what treatment is being given, it is almost impossible for his assessments of its efficacy to be impartial.

(b) *Types of control groups.*

- A no-treatment-group study is likely to be confounded because of the placebo effect in the treatment group, even if the treatment is inactive.

- Placebo: the control group receives an inert, dummy treatment which is indistinguishable from the treatment under study.

- A low-dose group: for the situation when a placebo group can not be used because of ethical issues.

- A group treated with a standard current therapy.

- 'Gold Standard' treatment group receiving the best current therapy.

- Historical controls, where the treatment group is compared with results obtained in previous 'similar' patients, are unreliable. The controls may well be significantly different than the current treatment group. The general management of patients with the condition in question may be different, the prognosis may be different, the natural history of the disease may be different, the state of nutrition may be different, the current patients may be more knowledgeable or may have been diagnosed earlier, and so on.

### 3. Randomization.

(a) *Random allocation to groups.*
- Randomization is used to ensure that the allocation of patients to the groups is independent of the characteristics of the patient. All patients have the same chance of being assigned to either intervention.
- If patients were allocated to groups by the investigator, it is impossible to exclude the possibility that, albeit unconsciously, the allocation is affected by patient factors that may influence the trial outcome, e.g. low-risk patients may be allocated to the treatment group. Randomization removes any chance of allocation bias.
- It is highly desirable that the treatment and control groups are similar with regard to factors that might affect outcome. Randomization, however, does not guarantee that this will be the case, although it does guarantee that differences will only occur by chance. For instance, there may be more females in one group than in the other, or the average age or the average weight of patients in the groups may be significantly different.
- Stratified randomization should therefore be used for factors that are believed to significantly influence the outcome.

(b) *Random sample of population.*
- If the results of a trial are to be generalizable, it is also important to ensure that the patients entering the trial are a random sample from the population of interest. Studies based on hospital admissions, for example, may not be generalizable to all patients with a particular disease since the types of patients admitted to different hospitals is variable, depending on factors like the particular hospital's catchment population, reputation, facilities, and so on.
- There is a better chance of detecting a treatment effect if there is little variability between the subjects. Restriction may be used to achieve this uniformity – e.g. by using only patients of a similar age, or a similar weight or similar severity of disease, etc. However, the danger here is that the more uniform the sample, the less generalizable are the results. Trials should investigate a sufficiently large sample of the population that the treatment will be used in.

(c) *Methods.*
- The three commonly used methods of randomization into groups are simple, restricted (or block) and stratified. They can be applied to parallel groups, cross-over or matched-pairs design trials.
- The methods of randomization are discussed further in the topic 'Randomization'.

### 4. Blinding.

(a) *Importance.*
- Bias may occur when either the investigator or the subject knows which treatment is being given. The investigator's observations and judgements

may become less objective and the patient's responses may become more positive or more negative depending on whether or not he is in the active treatment arm of the study.

- Therefore, clinical trials should use the maximum degree of blindness that is possible, so that patients or both patients and investigators are unaware of what treatment has been given.

(b) *Methods of blindness.*

- Double-blind means that neither the patient nor the investigator is aware of the treatment. This is the most desirable method to prevent assessment and response biases. However, in several fields, such as surgery, it may be impossible to run a double-blind study.
- In a single-blind trial, only the patient is unaware of the treatment.
- In a triple-blind trial, patient, investigator and also the data-monitoring body are unaware of the treatment group.
- The double dummy technique is used for drug trials comparing two active treatments, e.g. each patient receives one of the active tablets and a dummy tablet that looks like the alternative active tablet.
- In open trials, the investigators and patients know what treatment each patient is getting.

(c) *Randomization in a double-blind trial.*

- The most practical method of doing this is to use a series of consecutively numbered sealed opaque envelopes, each containing a treatment specification.
- For stratified randomization, it is necessary to use two or more sets of envelopes.

5. **Unblinding.**

(a) *Situations when blindness must be broken.*

- If the patient experiences symptoms or signs that may indicate an adverse reaction to the active treatment or if there is a significant deterioration in his/her medical condition, the blindness of the study must be broken.

(b) *Managing unblinding.*

- 'Breaking the code' should always be allowed for in the planning stage of the trial. The criteria for unblinding should be listed before the trial starts.
- The investigators should always be able to have emergency access to the randomization schedule.
- Treatment should be stopped and the patient withdrawn from the study.
- The code should be broken.
- The patient should receive the appropriate medical treatment.
- A formal safety monitoring committee should review the incident and make recommendations, if necessary.

## Observational studies

- The purpose of an observational study is to look for an association between a cause and an effect, between an exposure to a risk factor and the development of a particular disease.

- Observational studies are particularly relevant in epidemiology which is the branch of medicine that deals with the incidence, cause and prevention of disease.
- When looking for a link, for example, between smoking and lung cancer, investigators cannot use the classical tools of experimental research – they cannot randomize patients into a control group or a treatment group in order to confirm or refute a hypothesis, for obvious reasons. They must use other methods. They can observe a situation and analyse and interpret it, but they cannot intervene. Because subjects cannot be controlled or randomized, many observational studies are fraught with problems of bias.

## Case–control study

### 1. Definition.

- The retrospective case–control study starts with the identification of a group of individuals with the disease or condition of interest (cases) and a group of individuals without the disease (controls).
- The two groups are then compared with respect to their previous exposure to the risk factor or factors. A greater degree of exposure in the cases than in the controls suggests that the factor might be causally related to the disease.

### 2. Advantages and disadvantages.

- These studies can be carried out more speedily and cheaply than cohort studies, and they are particularly useful for rare diseases.
- However, difficulties and biases can occur at several points in the procedure, particularly when selecting controls.

### 3. Methods.

(a) *Selection of cases.*
- It is important to try to admit patients into the study at the same fixed point in the natural history of the disease, otherwise considerable bias will ensue.
- Often, only newly diagnosed patients are admitted, though even this is a variable feast, some patients being diagnosed earlier than others (lead time bias).

(b) *Selection of controls.*
- As in experimental studies, controls should be as similar to cases as possible, though without having the disease in question.
- The control may be another patient in the same hospital with another diagnosis. However, the risk factor may be linked to other diseases as well as the one under investigation, e.g. smoking may be associated with cardiac disease, stroke, gastrointestinal disease, respiratory disease as well as lung cancer. This may lead to an underestimation of the link.
- Alternatively, healthy subjects in the community may be selected but there may be difficulties in identifying a group with comparable characteristics to the cases.
- It may be helpful to match each case individually with a control rather than take a large random sample from the control population.

- It may also be possible to have more than one control per case if necessary. The two variables most frequently used for matching are age and gender.

4. **Other potential biases.**

(a) *Recall bias.*
   - Cases may be more likely to find stronger associations with the risk factors having had the time and the inclination to think of possible reasons for their problems.

(b) *Unreliable memories.*
   - In a retrospective study, much of the evidence depends on the possibly unreliable memories of the subjects.

(c) *Unreliable records.*
   - In many studies evidence may have to be elicited from notoriously unreliable hospital records.

(d) *Interview bias.*
   - It is acknowledged that different interviewers may obtain different information from the same patient.

# Cohort study

1. **Definition.**

- The prospective cohort study starts with the identity and examination of a group of subjects (the cohort) who are then followed up over a period of time looking for the development of a disease or other specified end-point.

2. **Advantages and disadvantages.**

(a) *Advantages.*
   - Cohort studies can be used to investigate the aetiology of a disease, e.g. diet and cardiovascular disease, or the prognosis of a disease, e.g. diet following myocardial infarction.
   - Because the study is prospective, data should be more accurate and reliable than in case–control studies. Thus, cohort studies should have major advantages over case–control studies.

(b) *Disadvantages.*
   - However, a cohort study usually requires that a large number of patients is followed up for a long period of time so that a sufficient number of subjects will develop the outcome of interest. They are therefore relatively inefficient and expensive, particularly when studying rare outcomes.

3. **Methods.**

- Subjects are classified at the beginning of the study into two (or more) groups, one exposed (e.g. cigarette smoker) and the other not exposed (non-smoker).
- At the end of the study the subgroups can be compared with respect to exposure to risk factors and disease outcome.

- In the simplest type of study the results can be summarized and compared in a $2 \times 2$ table (disease plus or minus versus exposure plus or minus, [see Chi squared and Fisher's exact test, p. 140]).

### 4. *Potential biases.*

- Subjects may be lost to follow-up during a long cohort study. This may lead to bias if the reason for loss of contact is related to the risk factors or the outcomes. A large loss to follow-up may significantly affect the validity of the results.
- Exposed subjects may reduce, while other subjects might increase, their exposure to the risk factors, e.g. by giving up or starting smoking.
- A change of occupation may reduce or increase exposure to, for example, asbestos.
- If the investigators are aware of the subject's group they may investigate exposed subjects more closely, so that 'surveillance bias' occurs.

## Cross-sectional study

### 1. *Methods.*

- In a cross-sectional study all the subjects are contacted or surveyed just once and at about the same time, usually by means of a questionnaire.
- The subjects may be a random sample of a defined population such as general practitioners or patients presenting with arthritis, etc.

### 2. *Advantages and disadvantages.*

- They may be designed to examine associations between risk factors and diseases. But since they do not examine temporal relationships, they may not be able to distinguish cause from effect. Therefore, they do not usually provide an insight into disease aetiology.
- They are a much better source of descriptive information, particularly about the prevalence rate of a disease or condition.

### 3. *Potential biases.*

- Non-response in cross-sectional surveys can be a major problem. There are likely to be important differences between the people who respond to surveys and the people who do not respond (volunteer bias), which may have a major impact on the results of the study. For example, responders may be healthier or older or more altruistic-minded or females. Hence the subjects responding to a survey may not be representative of the subjects invited to take part in it. Hence it may not be possible to extrapolate the results to the population under review.

## Further reading

Altman DG. Designing research. In: Altman DG, (ed). *Practical Statistics For Medical Research.* London: Chapman and Hall. 1991; pp. 74–106.

Bland M. The design of experiments. In: Bland M, (ed). *An Introduction to Medical Statistics.* Oxford: Oxford Medical Publication, 1995; pp. 5–25.

Daly LE, Bourke GJ. Epidemiological and clinical research methods. In: Daly LE, Bourke GJ, (eds). *Interpretation and Uses of Medical Statistics.* Oxford: Blackwell Science Ltd, 2000; pp. 143–201.

## Related topics of interest

Conducting clinical trials, p. 44; Randomization, p. 40; Medical research as part of post-graduate training, p. 1; Research process, p. 6.

# RANDOMIZATION

*YinHua Zhang, Fang Gao Smith*

The essence of many clinical trials is the comparison of groups of patients who receive different treatments. One of the fundamental principles of experimental design is that the patients are allocated to the treatment groups on a random basis.

## Objectives

**1. To prevent bias.** Random allocation gives all patients the same chance of receiving each treatment and is independent of the characteristics of the patients – in other words, it is carried out in an unbiased way.

(a) *Parallel-group studies.* In a parallel-group study, one group of patients receives one treatment, a second group receives the second treatment, and so on, if more than two treatments are being compared. Allocation of patients to the different treatments must be randomized against between-patient variations.

(b) *Cross-over studies.* In a cross-over study, each patient receives each treatment, on different occasions, with a sufficient time interval between treatments for the effect of one treatment to have worn off before the next is given. The order in which the treatments are given must be randomized against within-patient variations.

**2. The basis of statistical tests.** Statistical methods are based on what is expected to happen in random samples from populations with specified characteristics.

## Methods

**1. Simple randomization.** This method is probably the most common randomization procedure in practice, though it may not always be the best choice.

(a) *Tossing a coin.* For example, heads is treatment A, tails is treatment B.

(b) *Table of random numbers.*
- The numbers in the table are independent so that they are all random in any direction. Therefore, one can start from any number in any row or column.
- To assign a random number to the sample, one can make odd numbers indicate one treatment and even numbers the other for a parallel-group study; or randomly assign the two treatments A and B in an order of A–B or B–A in a cross-over study.
- These tables can be found in standard statistics books or a random number can be generated on a computer.

(c) *Disadvantages of simple randomization.*
- In trials of fewer than 100 patients, simple randomization may too easily result in seriously unequal treatment numbers.
- The method can not be recommended for multicentre trials because, even when treatment numbers are balanced over the trial as a whole, patients may be unequally allocated between treatments at individual hospitals.

- After simple randomization, other features, such as gender or age, can occur more frequently in one group than the other. For example, if five adult men are chosen in group A and five young girls are assigned to group B in a parallel study, the analysis will be flawed.

2. **Restricted (or block) randomization.** This is also called 'equal-numbers randomization' because it guarantees that numbers allocated to each treatment are equal after each 'block' of patients.

(a) *An example.* If two treatments (A or B) are to be given to a total of 32 patients, the randomization could be based on using 8 blocks of 4 patients.

(b) *Size of block and number of combinations.* Each block of 4 comprises different combinations of two A and two B treatments. With blocks of 4 there are six possible combinations of the two treatments:

(1) AABB      (2) ABBA      (3) ABAB
(4) BBAA      (5) BAAB      (6) BABA

Each combination is therefore given a number from one to six.

(c) *Using a random number table.* The order of the blocks is selected randomly by using a column or row in a random number table, accepting numbers from 1 to 6 and ignoring the numbers 7, 8, 9 and 0. The random sequence of treatments is then transferred to sealed, numbered envelopes so that the investigator giving the treatment is blinded.

(d) *Interspersed blocks.* The blocks of 4 should be interspersed with blocks of 2 or 6 so that the investigator is unable to deduce what treatment every fourth patient is going to receive.

3. **Stratified randomization.** This method ensures that each of the study groups receiving different treatments will have similar characteristics such as age or sex.

- This is achieved by preparing separate block randomizations for each subgroup, e.g. one for males and one for females or one for patients under 65 and one for patients over 65, etc.
- It is particularly important to ensure there is balance between the groups with regard to factors that are known to be of direct prognostic importance in a clinical trial, such as tumour size, tumour spread, lymph node involvement, etc. This will considerably increase the precision of the data analysis.

## Minimization method

Although minimization is a non-random method, it may be an acceptable method of allocation between small groups when there are several prognostic factors involved in the trial.

1. **Method.** The first patient to enter the trial is given a treatment at random. The treatment given to each subsequent patient is the one which results in a better balance between the groups with regard to the variables of interest.

*Worked example:*

(a) *Experiment.* The effect of cardiopulmonary bypass at 28°C or 37°C on cerebral blood flow.

(b) *Characteristics of the first 13 patients in the study.* See *Table 1.*

**Table 1.** Characteristics of the first 13 patients in a clinical trial using minimization to allocate treatments

|  |  | 28°C ($n=7$) | 37°C ($n=6$) |
|---|---|---|---|
| Age | ≤50 | 3 | 4 |
|  | >50 | 4 | 2 |
| Gender | Male | 5 | 3 |
|  | Female | 2 | 3 |
| Types of surgery | Valves | 4 | 4 |
|  | Coronary artery bypass grafting (CABG) | 3 | 2 |
| Previous stroke | Yes | 2 | 1 |
|  | No | 5 | 5 |

(c) *Characteristics of the new recruitment.* A male patient, 64 years old, who had a stroke 2 years ago, undergoing coronary artery bypass grafting surgery is the next patient to be recruited onto the trial. Which treatment should he have?

(d) *Calculate imbalance in patient characteristics. Table 2* lists the numbers of patients with this patient's characteristics already in the two treatment groups: 28°C = 14, 37°C = 8.

**Table 2.** Calculation of the overall imbalances in patient characteristics relevant to the recruitment of a 64-year-old male patient who has had a stroke and is scheduled for CABG

|  |  | 28°C ($n=7$) | 37°C ($n=6$) |
|---|---|---|---|
| Age | >50 | 4 | 2 |
| Gender | Male | 5 | 3 |
| Types of surgery | Coronary artery bypass grafting | 3 | 2 |
| Previous stroke | Yes | 2 | 1 |
|  | **Total** | **14** | **8** |

(e) *Decision on the new patient's allocation.* As the aim is to have the two groups as similar as possible, the preferable treatment for the new patient is that with the smaller total (37°C).

(f) *Decision on future patients' allocation.* The above process (a to d) should be repeated until the totals for the two treatments are the same, then the choice should be made using simple randomization (e.g. random number table).

**2. Disadvantage.** One difficulty with the method is that it requires details of all patients previously entered into the trial to be available before allocation can be made.

## Further reading

Altman DG. *Practical Statistics for Medical Research.* London: Chapman and Hall, 1991.

Armitage P, Berry G. *Statistical Methods in Medical Research.* Oxford: Blackwell Scientific Publications, 1994.

Elston RC, Johnson WD. *Essentials of Biostatistics.* Essentials of Medical Education Series, Philadelphia: FA Davis Company, 1987.

Pocock SJ. *Clinical Trials: A practical approach.* Chichester: Wiley, 1983.

## Related topic of interest

Conducting clinical trials, p. 44.

# CONDUCTING CLINICAL TRIALS

*Alan Casson*

---

Clinical trials are the most sophisticated form of clinical research and they can give clear and direct answers to many research questions. The principles of the design of experimental and observational studies have been discussed in the topic 'Research design' (p. 31). This topic deals with the practical aspects of conducting clinical trials.

## History

Current concepts of trial design and methodology have evolved following the report of a randomized clinical trial which demonstrated the efficacy of streptomycin compared to bed rest in the treatment of tuberculosis over 50 years ago. Since then, clinical trials have been utilized in virtually all areas of medical and surgical practice.

## Protocol of a clinical trial

**1. Definition.** A protocol is a formal document outlining the proposed procedures for carrying out the study. It itemizes every aspect, from the hypothesis, through selection of the study groups, their treatment, the collection of data and their analysis.

**2. Importance.** The protocol should be so comprehensive that, in the event of the unexpected demise of the principal investigator, any intelligent replacement could continue it using only the protocol.

- Such a protocol is not only for the use of the investigators themselves, but also the monitoring study committee and the local ethics committee.
- Furthermore, the protocol greatly simplifies the writing up of the publication.

**3. Format.** The main features of the protocol include:

(a) *Title page.* This page includes the title of the study, the name and address (phone, e-mail, fax) of the principal investigator and the date of the manuscript.

(b) *Background and hypothesis.*
- This defines the specific research question and develops the hypothesis, which is a statement about the assumed relationship between the variables or the outcomes to be tested.
- This should include a review of the relevant background and current state of knowledge related to the clinical problem and justify the need for the trial.

(c) *Study design.* The type of study proposed should be described. The principles of research design are discussed further in the topic 'Research design', p. 31.

(d) *Materials and methodology.*
- This is the most important section of the protocol. The interventions and methods to be used must be described in detail.
- This part of the protocol is discussed further in the next section of this topic.

(e) *Data collection and handling.*

- Research data may be collected in various ways, which are described in detail in the topic 'Data collection' (p. 64).
- A data handling form is designed for each patient. Relevant data are collected by defined individuals (e.g. clinical trial nurses, study physicians) and recorded on paper ('hard' copy) and in electronic (computer) format.
- Data security is essential to prevent unauthorized access to personal medical information.

(f) *Statistical analysis.* The statistical considerations of a clinical trial are discussed further below.

(g) *References.*

(h) *Summary.* In a complicated trial with a lengthy protocol, it is always helpful to provide a short summary with a schematic flow chart which can be either listed after the title page or at the end of the protocol.

## Methodology

### 1. Ethical approval and informed consent.

- All clinical trials in the UK and in most other Western countries require approval by an appropriate ethics committee. The use of human subjects makes informed consent mandatory.
- Even if only the medical records are involved, appropriate safeguards are needed for data confidentiality, the protection of privacy and the prevention of unauthorized access.

### 2. Inclusion and exclusion criteria.
The trial protocol should clearly identify the target patient population, with well-defined clinically applicable inclusion and exclusion criteria.

- The more stringent the inclusion and exclusion criteria, the more homogeneous the sample will be. This may be useful in a study with a small sample but may mean that results and conclusions of the study will be less generalizable to the population as a whole.
- In larger studies it is better not to be too restrictive with inclusion and exclusion criteria.

### 3. Evaluation and endpoint measurements.

(a) *Evaluation and assessment.* These include clinical assessments by the patients (e.g. pain visual analogue scales) and by clinicians (e.g. stages of cancer, or adverse events), routine laboratory investigations (e.g. haematology, clinical chemistry) and designed investigations (e.g. measurements of cytokines).

(b) *Endpoint measurements.* These are quantitative measurements or qualitative observations required by the aims of the study.
  - Primary endpoints answer the main question, whilst
  - Secondary endpoints refer to other interesting clinical aspects of the trial.
  - If the clinical relevant endpoint can not be found directly a surrogate endpoint is usually used.

(c) *Intervals of evaluations and measurements.* The decision on how frequently the measurements should be taken depends on factors such as pharmacokinetics (e.g. the half-life of a drug or enzyme) or the changes expected in the patient's clinical condition, etc.

(d) *Precision and accuracy.* The precision and the accuracy of measurements must be described in detail including coefficient of variation, standard deviation of the measurement, correlation coefficient, limits of agreement, etc. (See topic 'Measurements', p. 68, for further details.)

**4. Protocol deviations.** It is necessary to state how to deal with patients who deviate from the protocol and how much modification of drug dose is permitted within the protocol in patients who respond abnormally or who experience minor unwanted effects of the drug.

## Statistical considerations

**1. Sample size.** An estimate of the number of subjects needed for the study is an integral part of the design process, and should be determined in consultation with the statistician.

- Sample size and power calculations (the probability of detecting an event) depend on the study design, statistical analysis and the significance levels that are set (see topic 'Sample size and power', p. 50).
- As a general rule, the larger the expected difference between the groups, the smaller is the sample size required to detect the difference.
- The more groups that are studied, the greater the sample size needed.
- In the cross-over design, each patient is his or her own control, therefore within-patient variation is reduced. Hence, a cross-over trial needs a smaller number of patients to detect a given effect with a given power.

**2. Interim analyses.**

(a) *Definition.* An interim analysis compares the groups while the trial is still in progress to determine whether the trial should be stopped for patient safety (adverse events) or because of a demonstrated benefit to patients in one arm of the study.

(b) *Methods*
- The pre-planned, restricted number of interim analyses to be performed should be specified in the protocol.
- The interim analyses should be performed by a blinded and independent staff from a data and safety monitoring committee.
- The endpoint may be re-defined statistically after an interim analysis.
- Interim analyses are universally applied in large, multi-centre trials, and they are of particular importance in survival studies, which often continue for several years.

(c) *α-adjustment*
- Repeated comparisons will increase the chance for type I error (the finding of a significant difference between groups purely by chance). In order to

reduce this error, $\alpha$-adjustment is used to determine the $P$-value at which the trial should be stopped.

- $\alpha$-adjustment may be calculated by dividing the pre-determined $P$-value (conventionally 0.05) by the pre-planned number of interim analyses (Bonferroni-adjustment). Hence if five interim analyses are proposed, the $P$-value must be reduced to $<0.01$.

3. *Intention to treat analysis.*

(a) *Protocol violation.* A problem commonly seen in trials is that some of the subjects will not receive the full course of treatment allocated to them. Typical reasons for this are: patient withdrawal because of side effects, poor compliance or loss to follow up. As a result, there will be a smaller number of patients who have actually received the study treatment. This situation may be managed by per protocol analysis or by intention to treat analysis.

(b) *Per protocol analysis*
- Per protocol analysis only analyses the data collected from patients who actually adhered to the protocol and ignores the patients who have been randomized to receive the study treatment or placebo but did not receive it.
- Per protocol analysis may result in bias, particularly if the allocated treatment has adverse effects or is ineffective. It will then over-estimate the true benefit and under-estimate adverse effects of the treatment.

(c) *Intention to treat analysis*
- Intention to treat analysis is based on the data collected from all groups as randomized (i.e. according to the intention to treat, rather than what actually happened).
- This is the only safe method to deal with all situations related to protocol violation.
- Intention to treat analysis must be considered the main analysis if per protocol analysis is also performed.

# Drug development studies: Phases I–IV

After extensive testing in the laboratory and in animals, newly developed drugs are tested in formal human studies. Trials involving humans are divided into four phases.

1. **Phase I studies** are usually carried out in 25–50 healthy volunteers. However, toxicity trials of oncological drugs would use volunteers with advanced disease and malignancy. Phase I trials are designed to determine the basic pharmokinetic data, the maximum tolerated dose and the optimum dose of the drug.

2. **Phase II studies** are usually carried out in 100–200 patients with disease who might benefit from the drug. They aim to establish the dose–response relationship, evaluate the efficacy of the agent and estimate the rate of adverse events.

Both phase I and phase II clinical trials are usually open and unblinded, both patient and investigator being aware of the exact nature of the drug.

3. **Phase III studies** are the formal clinical trials that assess the effectiveness and safety of the agent in several thousand patients. The new drug is compared with a

placebo or a standard treatment in studies involving controls, randomization and blinding of both investigators and patients.

*4. Phase IV studies* are carried out in the general population after the new drug has been approved. They focus on long-term follow-up (post-market surveillance) of patients receiving the drug or intervention. This phase does not require controls, randomization or blinding and allows for the determination of safety and efficacy over an extended period of time.

## Multicentre clinical trials

*1. Advantages.* The principal advantages of multicentre trials are:

- access to a greater sample size;
- accelerated recruitment;
- increased study power.

Although most such studies are prospective, randomized and controlled, access to pooled data from participating centres may permit retrospective studies to be performed in selected situations.

*2. Disadvantages.* Potential difficulties of multicentre trials relate to trial coordination, inconsistency of data and interventions in the various participating centres, and initial difficulties with obtaining uniform ethics committee approval.

## Administrative structure

- The clinical trial should be organized as simply as possible, with a clearly defined study leader (principal investigator).
- It is essential to identify the responsibilities of study team members to avoid duplication and overlap of duties.

## Funding

- A realistic budget should be developed early in the study design.
- Several funding opportunities exist for clinical research, locally, regionally, nationally and internationally (see topic 'Grant application', p. 60).
- It is important to ensure that the objectives of the funding agency are comparable with those of the study, and therefore the agency regulations, policies and terms of reference should be studied with care before an application is submitted.
- It is important to ensure that no overlap exists between agencies funding a specific project.

# Further reading

Kahn CR. Picking a research problem. The critical decision. *The New England Journal of Medicine* 1994; **330**: 1530–1533.

Rusch VW. Thoracic surgery clinical trials: Y2K and beyond. *Annals of Thoracic Surgery* 1999; **68**: 2–3.

Simpson PM, Spratt JA, Spratt JS. Statistical methods in cancer research. *Journal of Surgical Oncology* 2001; **76**: 201–223.

Troidl H, Spitzer WO, McPeek B. *Principles and Practice of Research. Strategies for Surgical Investigators,* 2nd edn. New York: Springer-Verlag, 1991.

## Related topics of interest

Data collection, p. 64; Grant application, p. 60; Measurements, p. 68; Medical research as part of post-graduate training, p. 1; Randomization, p. 40; Research ethics committees, p. 55; Research design, p. 31; Sample size and power, p. 50; Systematic review and meta-analysis. p. 167; Volunteer studies, p. 23.

# SAMPLE SIZE AND POWER

*Craig Jackson, Fang Gao Smith*

Clinical trials often involve the comparison of a new treatment with an established treatment (or a placebo) in a sample of patients, and the differences between the two treatment groups is analysed using a hypothesis test. It is important that the sample size is large enough to detect a treatment effect, at a given significance level, if there is one. If the sample size is too small there is the likelihood that a type II error will occur.

## Types of error in hypothesis testing

The two types of error that can occur when using hypothesis tests are summarized in *Table 1*.

**Table 1.** The types of errors associated with hypothesis tests ($H_0$ = null hypothesis)

|  | Decision to accept $H_0$ | Decision to reject $H_0$ |
|---|---|---|
| $H_0$ true | Correct decision | Type I error (false positive) Probability $\alpha$ |
| $H_0$ false | Type II error (false negative) | Correct decision Probability $\beta$ |

1. ***Type I error.***

- A type I error occurs if the null hypothesis is rejected, i.e. a significant result is obtained, when the null hypothesis is in fact true.
- A type I error is a 'false-positive' result.
- The probability of making a type I error is denoted as $\alpha$.

2. ***Type II error.***

- A type II error occurs if the null hypothesis is accepted, i.e. an insignificant result is obtained, when the null hypothesis is in fact not true (the alternative hypothesis is true).
- A type II error is a 'false-negative' result.
- The probability of making a type II error is denoted as $\beta$.

## The importance of sample size

- In many published clinical trials, it is apparent that little consideration has been given to the appropriate sample size required to confirm or refute the investigators' hypotheses. The default sample size is sometimes far too small to detect anything but the most gross difference. A non-significant result is reported and a type II error may occur.
- On the other hand, a sample that is too large is an unnecessary waste of clinical resources and brings ethical issues, regarding patients' inconvenience and unnecessary discomfort, etc., into question.

- It is therefore essential to make an assessment of the optimal sample size required before starting an investigation and to report the sample size calculation in the subsequent paper.

## Factors affecting required sample size

In clinical trials involving, for example, the comparison of two independent groups, the sample size required depends on power, clinically worthwhile difference to be detected, standard deviation of the variable and the nominated significance level. These factors are interdependent so that it is possible to calculate any one of them given the others.

### 1. Power.

- Power is the probability that a study of a given size would detect as statistically significant a real difference of a given magnitude.
- It is generally recommended that the power of a clinical trial should be at least 80–90%.
- A high power means that there is a high chance of detecting a significant difference, if there is one, and a low chance of making a type II error. With a high power, if a result is non-significant, one can be reasonably sure, though not certain, that it is valid to accept the null hypothesis.
- Since the probability of not detecting a real difference between study groups is $\beta$ (i.e. the probability of a type II error), the probability of detecting a real difference (the power) is $1 - \beta$.

### 2. Minimum clinically worthwhile difference.

(a) *Hypothesized difference and sample size.*
  - If the difference between two treatments is large then relatively small samples are likely to produce a significant result. If the difference between treatments is small then much larger numbers are required.

(b) *Statistical significance and clinical significance.*
  - When differences are expected to be small, it becomes important to distinguish between statistical significance and clinical significance.
  - The investigator needs to define the minimum difference between the groups that he is going to consider clinically relevant. For example, suppose that a new bronchodilator is believed to cause a real increase in tidal volume of 10 ml in patients with chronic bronchitis. The standard deviation of tidal volume in this population is likely to be considerably higher than this figure. It would be possible, however, given a huge sample, to demonstrate the real increase, but the exercise would be very expensive and very pointless because with such a small (but statistically significant) difference, the drug would be of little clinical consequence.
  - Given a large enough sample, any difference, no matter how small and trivial, can be made statistically significant.
  - Hence, experience and judgement are needed when deciding the minimum treatment effect that is going to be of value to patients and which therefore justifies the time, effort and finance required to investigate it.

### 3. Standard deviation.

- The larger the standard deviations of the two groups relative to the minimal clinically important difference to be detected, the larger the sample size that is going to be required; the smaller the standard deviations, the smaller the sample size required.
- The ratio of the minimal clinically important difference to the standard deviation is referred to as the standardized difference and is used in the Altman nomogram.

### 4. The estimated SD. At the start of many investigations, an estimate of the standard deviation may not be readily available. There are several approaches to this problem:

- Perform a pilot study.
- Start the trial with the intention of estimating the likely standard deviation from the first patients.
- Use the standard deviation found in the investigator's own previous trials of a similar kind.
- Use the standard deviation quoted in similar trials or in similar patients in similar circumstances reported in the literature.

### 5. Significance level.

- The significance level, $\alpha$, has an important bearing on the sample size required. If the significance level chosen is 0.01 rather than 0.05, a much larger sample size will be required to avoid a $\beta$ error, whereas if $\alpha$ is 0.1 then a much smaller sample size will be adequate, though there is then an increased risk of making a type I error.
- There is a reciprocal relationship between $\alpha$ and $\beta$ – as the nominated $\alpha$ decreases the chances of a $\beta$ error increases and *vice versa*. In other words, for a given sample size, if $\alpha$ is 0.01 rather than 0.05, there is a smaller probability of making a type I error but greater probability of making type II error. An $\alpha$ value of 0.05 implies that 1 trial in 20 will produce a type I error purely by chance.
- As a rule of thumb the probability of a type II error of a study should be approximately 4 times the significance level chosen. For example, if the significance level is 5%, the power should be at least 80%. If the significance level is 1%, the power should be 95%.

## Calculating the sample size

Mathematical methods are available for estimating the sample sizes required for every type of clinical trial, with both categorical and continuous data, comparisons of means and proportions, one, two or more groups, paired and unpaired samples, groups of equal or unequal sizes. However, the formulae used are complex and for many investigators, the guidance of a statistician would be essential.

Two alternative approaches are available for medical investigators with limited mathematical knowledge.

### 1. The Altman normogram.

(a) *Advantages.* The normogram is a simple and elegant idea that can be applied to categorical and continuous data including paired and unpaired samples and groups of unequal sizes.

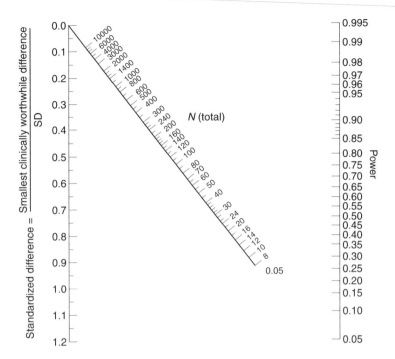

Figure 1. A normogram

(b) *Using the normogram.*
- The normogram (*Figure 1*) relates standardized difference (left scale), significance level (middle scale) and power (right scale). In the next section, the normogram will be used to find the sample size required for a two-independent-group comparison of a continuous measurement.
- Let the standardized difference (smallest clinically worthwhile difference/SD) = 1.05, the significance level = 0.05 and the power = 0.85. A straight line is drawn between 1.05 on the standardized difference scale and 0.85 on the power scale. The line passes through $n = 30$ on the 0.05 significance scale. Therefore, 15 patients in each group will be sufficient to detect the smallest clinically important difference between the two groups with power of 0.85 at a significance level of 0.05.

## 2. *Computers.*

- Investigator-friendly computer software programs are available that can calculate sample sizes quickly and automatically.
- Also, several pages on the world wide web are dedicated to assisting investigators with automatic sample size calculations.

## Further reading

Altman DG. Statistics and ethics in medical research. III How large a sample? *British Medical Journal*. 1980; **281:** 1336–1338.

Altman DG. Clinical trials. In: Altman DG (Ed). *Practical Statistics for Medical Research*. London, Chapman & Hall, 1991, pp. 440–474.

## Related topics of interest

Choice of statistical tests, p. 164; Research design, p. 31; Research process, p. 6; Conducting clinical trials, p. 44; Principles of statistical analysis – estimation and hypothesis testing, p. 99.

# RESEARCH ETHICS COMMITTEES

*Danny McAuley*

The purpose of a research ethics committee is to consider the ethics of proposed research projects which will involve human subjects within the National Heath Service (NHS).

## General information

1. ***Research ethics committees have two major roles.***

- to protect subjects from unethical research.
- to encourage research.

2. ***They bring two further benefits.***

- They protect the research from the consequences of personal enthusiasm.
- They protect the reputation of the institution where research is carried out.

3. ***Research ethical committees function at two levels.***

(a) *The local research ethics committee (LREC)*
   - An LREC is responsible for any NHS body within a given geographical area.
   - The LREC and its members are independent of the NHS bodies to which they provide ethical advice. An LREC is normally made up of 8–12 members with medical, nursing and lay representation. The health professionals include those primarily involved in clinical care and those experienced in research. The members are independent of the groups from which they are drawn and are appointed as individuals with relevant experience.

(b) *The multi-centre research ethics committee (MREC)*
   - MRECs were established in 1997 in an attempt to simplify the process of organizing multi-centre research. There is an MREC in each English region, and one each in Scotland and Wales.
   - MREC approval is required if a study is to be carried out in five or more centres. Following MREC approval an LREC fast track subcommittee also reviews the research protocol within 3 weeks with comments limited to local issues alone.

## Responsibility for research

1. ***Ethics committee approval.*** An ethical committee must be consulted for research involving:

- NHS patients, including access to medical records
- foetal material and In Vitro Fertilization (IVF) involving NHS patients
- the recently dead in NHS premises
- the use of NHS facilities.

2. ***Department of Research and Development.*** All research in the NHS is conducted under the auspices of the Department of Research and Development, as required by the Research Governance Framework of the Department of Health. No

research should be started until the project has been registered, reviewed and approved by the local Department of Research and Development on behalf of the Trust. The Department is briefed to take into account all relevant guidance and advice given by the Ethics Committee.

### 3. *Legal liability.*

- It is important to emphasize that researchers are not absolved of responsibility by obtaining ethical approval. Legal liability remains principally with the researcher and the NHS body in which the research is undertaken.

## Issues for the ethics committee

In deciding if a research proposal is ethical the ethics committee needs to consider:

- the scientific merit of the proposal
- the effect on the health of the research subjects
- the potential hazards, including discomfort or distress
- the experience of the researcher
- the degree of supervision during the project
- the procedure for informed consent
- the information sheet to be provided.

## Recruitment of subjects

- Participation must be voluntary: this is particularly important if subjects are drawn from a dependent group such as medical students or patients.
- It must be made clear that refusal to participate will not result in any disadvantage.
- Furthermore, subjects must be free to withdraw at any time and do not need to offer any reason for not taking part nor for withdrawing.

## Volunteers' health status

Researchers are responsible for determining that volunteers have a health status which does not preclude involvement. With the subject's permission, their General Practitioner should be informed of participation in a study. The patient should not be considered for a study if there is refusal to allow such contact.

## Consent

- Written informed consent is normally mandatory for all research and consent should be documented in the patient's medical records.
- Central to obtaining valid informed consent is the provision of a patient information sheet explaining the planned research in detail to be kept including recruitment, confidentiality, explanation of lack of personal benefit in non-therapeutic research, indemnity and contacts, including whom to contact in the event of concerns regarding the conduct of the study.
- Consent for an incompetent patient to take part in a clinical trial, e.g. a sedated critically ill patient in intensive care or unconscious patient, requires specific considerations. No person, even the next-of-kin, is able to give valid consent for another adult. The ethics committee needs to be satisfied that proceeding without prospective consent is ethically acceptable.

- This problem highlights the potential difficulties that ethics committees face, striking a balance between ensuring that research is ethically acceptable and avoiding obstruction of potentially valuable research which could improve patient care.
- To enter an incompetent patient into a clinical trial requires written authorisation from the researcher and the consultant in change of the patient's care, assent should be obtained from the next-of-kin and subsequently written informed (retrospective) consent obtained from the patient if he/she regains competence.
- The advantages of this approach were recently demonstrated in a large study examining a commonly used treatment for patients with severe head injury who are frequently unconscious. The ethics committee waived the need for informed consent and the study showed that the treatment was ineffective and possibly increased mortality. Without this ethics committee approval the study could not have been completed and a potentially harmful treatment would have continued to be used. Similarly, a delay occasioned by the need to obtain informed consent may delay a treatment which is potentially only useful if given early and therefore may itself affect the outcome of the study.

## Confidentiality

- Researchers must assure the ethics committee that:
  1. personal clinical information will remain confidential;
  2. that no unauthorized access will be allowed;
  3. no person will be identifiable from published results.
- With regard to epidemiological research using medical records, it may not be necessary to obtain consent from every individual. The ethics committee must be satisfied that this kind of research is conducted in accordance with data protection legislation and that the value of such a project outweighs the principle that individual consent should be required.
- Consent to have access to the medical records or to contact the subject should be obtained from the health professional responsible for the subject's care.

## Financial considerations

- Payment to subjects should be for expense, time and inconvenience incurred and not as an inducement to people to take part in studies against their judgement or to take part in several studies. Many subjects, however, may not be prepared to sacrifice the required time and suffer the inconvenience to take part in a study without adequate remuneration.
- This is a concept that ethics committees may fail to grasp. As with the issue of consent, it may be necessary to 'play the game' in that proposals will frequently be accepted as long as payment is described as 'expenses' regardless of whether this provides financial inducement or not.
- Clearly, money is an inducement to take part in research and, regardless of ethical approval, it is the ethical duty of the researcher not to allow a subject to take part in studies which may be potentially detrimental.
- Payment to the researcher is another aspect to consider. A researcher is unlikely to undertake a pharmaceutical-based study unless there is financial reward for the department. However, this must not influence the researcher's judgement in

the recruitment and treatment of subjects, which is the responsibility of the individual researcher rather than the ethics committee. Any personal payment to researchers themselves is inappropriate.

## Compensation

- NHS bodies will not offer indemnity for adverse events occurring as a result of a recognized risk of the research: however, if an adverse event occurs as a result of negligence the subject can claim for compensation through litigation.
- Pharmaceutical companies should provide compensation in the event of adverse events and the ethics committee will need to be satisfied that the company accepts responsibility for compensation.
- The ethics committee must be satisfied that the subjects are aware of all known risks and potential difficulties in obtaining compensation. This is a difficult area as there must be a balance between informing subjects and providing a litany of potential catastrophes likely to deter all subjects from even considering taking part in a research study.

## Drugs

- The ethics committee must be provided with assurances of the quality and stability of any drug to be administered. If a drug is to be used outside its Product Licence the ethics committee must be reassured that its use as part of a research study is safe.
- This may be done by obtaining details of the clinical trials exemption certificate.

## Therapeutic and non-therapeutic research

- Research is classified as either therapeutic or non-therapeutic.
- Therapeutic research carries the prospect of a direct benefit to the research subject, while non-therapeutic research, although potentially associated with collective benefit, is not expected to result in any direct benefit. This is a somewhat artificial division.
- There is a misconception that research studies are undertaken at the expense of present patients for the benefit of future patients. Given the frequent clinical uncertainty regarding current treatments and the substantial evidence that people do better in trials than during routine treatment, clinical care may be improved by inclusion in a research trial, whatever treatment group patients are assigned to.
- In essence, research may be regarded as controlled data collection in the setting of clinical uncertainty.

## Making an application

*1. Guidance.* Problems are minimized by presenting the proposal in the manner dictated by the ethics committee.

- Contact the committee chairperson for guidance on submissions. Obtain a copy of any such guidelines and follow them as closely as possible.
- It is particularly important to follow instruction regarding consent and financial details.
- It can be very useful to discuss the planned submission with a person who has made successful submissions to that ethics committee in the past.

2. *Statement of the reason for undertaking the study.* It is important to state clearly the reason for undertaking the study and, particularly in the case of non-therapeutic research, what the potential benefits of the results from the study might be.

3. *Patient information sheets.* Ethics committees frequently have major difficulties with patient information sheets.

- Most will have standard instructions for writing such information sheets requiring the inclusion of fully drafted paragraphs on the matters discussed above. These should be quoted verbatim.
- The ethics committee will frequently also have a standard consent form which should be reproduced.
- The information sheet must be written in clear, non-medical language that is understandable to a lay person. The potential risks must be honestly stated although every rare risk need not be described.
- If similar techniques have been previously used within a department, subjects may be reassured by providing the incidence (if any) of potential complications.

4. *Approval or rejection.*

- Ethics committees, given that they are made up of ordinary people, are idiosyncratic and a research protocol will be approved on one occasion, whereas a submission of a similar proposal will be rejected. This can be frustrating but it probably reflects the difficulties faced by the ethics committee.
- Most reasonable research proposals will be approved although, frequently this will involve considerable interchange between the researcher and the committee to deal with concerns about protocol. When replying to such concerns it is essential to reference your reply to each point raised by the ethics committee.
- If the ethics committee is insistent in its refusal to approve a protocol it is useful to clarify on what specialist advice their decision has been taken.
- It is worth remembering that the role of the ethics committee is to protect subjects involved in research and that the committee may have identified concerns which have not been previously recognized and which may be fully justified.

## Further reading

Alberti KGMM. Multicentre research ethics committees: has the cure been worse than the disease? *British Medical Journal* 2000; **320:**1157–1158.
Local Research Ethics Committees, Department of Health Report, 1992.
Narayan RK. Hypothermia for traumatic brain injury – a good idea proved ineffective *The New England Journal of Medicine* 2001; **344:** 8.

## Related topics of interest

Research process, p. 6; Writing up: case report, publications and thesis, p. 176; Conducting clinical trials, p. 44.

# GRANT APPLICATION

*Alan Casson*

Research requires money. Funding is obtained through the submission of a research grant application. This also serves to focus future research directions and, if successful, recognizes the quality of an individual's research efforts. However, many grant applications are unsuccessful and several applications and re-submissions are generally required in an increasingly competitive environment.

## Sources of research funding

There are three basic types of funding source.

*1. Peer-reviewed funds.* These are considered the most prestigious. There are two basic sources: publicly funded, either directly by the government or one of the research councils, or major charities such as the Wellcome Foundation. Nearly all of the available peer-reviewed granting bodies can be found on the internet.

*2. Industrial funds.* There are many companies with new drugs, devices, or other medical innovations who are dependent on finding academic investigators to take on projects on their behalf.

*3. Local institutional funds.* These are often the first funding a young researcher will receive to begin research.

## General outline of an application

An appropriate funding body must be selected, its policies and terms of reference studied, and instructions for grant submission followed in detail. The application should be written clearly and precisely, with no spelling or typographical errors. It is advisable to get the application reviewed by knowledgeable peers before formal submission to the granting body. There are a number of essential elements:

*1. An important question.* The question must either address an unmet clinical need, or it must address a fundamental biological mechanism. The best questions address both.

*2. A reasonable hypothesis.* The hypothesis should be developed against a background review of the literature. This need not be exhaustive, but should focus on the current state of knowledge and controversies in the area. Sufficient references should be cited, as it is likely that the reviewer, although knowledgeable, will not be directly involved in the specific area of research. The hypothesis should be:

- meaningful;
- original;
- plausible.

*3. Convincing preliminary data.* Nearly all peer-reviewed funding bodies require convincing preliminary data (usually funded by local institutional start-up grants) as evidence that the applicant has the ability to perform the studies.

4. **Ethical and biosafety approval.** Most funding bodies require institutions and the researcher to obtain ethical and biosafety approval for human, animal and laboratory studies.

5. **Convincing study methodology.** The proposed research should reflect the state of the art, and the grant application should show that you understand the proposed methodology thoroughly. The applicant(s) must provide evidence of ability to complete the proposed research.

6. **Budgets.**
- *Salaries* are usually the most expensive item in a research budget.
- *Other costs* include equipment, supplies, raw materials, animal care, manuscript preparation and travel, etc.
- *Overheads* are set by the institution and can range up to more than 100% on top of the direct costs. This is intended to cover the upkeep of the fabric of the building and the administration of the research.

## General notions

1. **Reputation.** There are three ways to establish a scientific reputation:
- Obtaining a research degree with an established supervisor and publishing papers;
- Presenting your work at scientific meetings;
- Building up appropriate 'collaborative networks'.

2. **Honesty.** Nobody will fund your research if they do not believe you are an honest scientist.

3. **Modesty.** A grant application that displays self-promotion is unlikely to attract a reviewer's favour. Do not diminish the contributions of other scientists or inflate your own.

4. **Performance.** There are three components:
- *Recruitment:* this must be met at a rate which ensures that the study is completed by the deadline.
- *Adherence:* the study must strictly adhere to the approved study protocol.
- *Documentation:* records must be completed as precisely as possible and the paperwork, such as informed consents, must be well maintained.

5. **Persistence.** Most peer-reviewed grants are not approved on the first review. If a grant application is rejected, it should be dealt with as for a rejected paper (see topic on Peer review).

## Special points concerning funding from industry

This is generally easier to obtain than peer-reviewed funding. The general outline of an application is the same: the only significant difference is that there is little emphasis on preliminary data. There are, however, several important extra points.

1. **Honesty and performance.** These are the attributes which companies most care about. For example, if you forget to record a blood pressure at 5 minutes after

some intervention, but recorded blood pressure at 1 and 10 minutes after, you must not interpolate a blood pressure at 5 minutes by averaging the values at 1 and 10 minutes.

**2. *The agreement.*** This will be a contract: you should price it at a level which will ensure that you can deliver a good product; industrial sponsors will gladly pay top price for top-quality clinical research.

**3. *Publishing.*** The final decision about what is published must remain exclusively at the discretion of the principal investigator. However, it is reasonable to grant the sponsor permission to review a manuscript, offer suggestions and request a certain day delay in publication if there are patent issues that need to be resolved prior to publication.

**4. *Potential conflicts of interest.***

- There is a natural desire to justify the sponsor's investment by obtaining a result favourable to the product. If the study is unfavourable or negative, the investigators may be put under pressure to simply not publish the results at all or only have a short discussion.
- Mixing consulting activity with industrial research can be a very effective way to obtain research funding. Potential sponsors often want an expert opinion early in the process of developing a new drug, device or technology. However, a conflict of interest can be created when the consulting relationship is converted into the relationship of a principal investigator to a sponsor. At this point, it is wise to cease any consulting relationship and establish a clean financial arrangement between the sponsor, your institute and yourself.
- It is unwise to have a financial interest in the sponsor's business.

## Local institutional funding

This is usually awarded only to promising individuals with a good idea, with none of the requirements for preliminary data and successful track record that are associated with peer-reviewed and industrial funding. However, this funding should be used as seed money to launch one's future funding.

## Some final points

**1. *Renewal.*** If a grant has been awarded, the granting body may have competitive mechanisms for its renewal. Criteria for successful renewal include the ability to demonstrate that the aims of the original application were met, within budget, and with evidence of productivity by publications and presentations.

**2. *Think one grant ahead.*** Always promise top-notch research, always deliver top-notch research, always request top rate for your work and always think one grant ahead.

**3. *Be passionate about your research.*** When you are successful, never forget today's success can not insulate you from failure in the future. When you fail, be confident that your honesty, humility, performance and persistence will certainly lead to future success.

**4. *Success begets funding, which begets more success.*** Researchers who do not have a successful track record are quickly identified and weeded out.

## Further reading

Kahn CR. Picking a research problem. The critical decision. *New England Journal of Medicine* 1994; **330:** 1530–1533.

Kron IL. Getting funded. *Journal of Thoracic and Cardiovascular Surgery* 2000; **119:** S26–S28.

Schwinn DA, DeLong ER, Shafer SL. Writing successful research proposals for medical science. *Anesthesiology* 1998; **88:** 1660–1666.

Troidl H, Spitzer WO, McPeek B. *Principles and Practice of Research. Strategies for Surgical Investigators,* 2nd edn, New York: Springer-Verlag, 1991.

## Related topics of interest

Conducting clinical trials, p. 44; Peer review, p. 185.

# DATA COLLECTION

*Aw Tar-Ching*

An essential part of research is the systematic, careful, and complete collection of relevant data that are then subjected to summary and analysis to yield answers or clues to research questions. Research data may be collected in various ways. In part this is dependent on the design and nature of the study.

## Methods of data collection

*1. Questionnaires.* A standardized questionnaire is the most commonly used method in epidemiological studies involving human volunteers.

(a) *Types of questionnaires.* Questionnaires can be self-administered or interviewer-administered.

- Self-administered questionnaires are completed by the study participants.
- In the interviewer-administered questionnaires, interviewers are trained to present the questions systematically to the study participants, and record their responses. The training of interviewers for epidemiological studies includes guidance on what clarification should be provided if a participant has a query regarding any of the questions. This is to ensure consistency in the explanations provided by the interviewers.

(b) *Questions.*

- Questions in epidemiological studies are often provided with a limited choice of answers, and the participants have to select the most appropriate answer (and tick the chosen 'box' on the questionnaire accordingly).
- In some instances, responders may be allowed to choose more than one response.
- Open-ended questions have space allocated for recording whatever response is provided. However, such responses are difficult to analyse without the introduction of some bias in interpretation, and are therefore less used in epidemiological research.

*2. Findings from clinical examination.* Clinical research may require that a trained clinician examines one or more specified target organ systems and records the findings.

(a) *Findings.* This may be a simple observation such as pulse rate or blood pressure, or determining the presence of, for example, a skin rash, enlarged liver or a cataract.

(b) *Standardization.* Even for relatively simple clinical observations such as blood pressure, the procedure must be standardized or else variations will occur between patients purely because of difference in the procedure used. Thus for blood pressure measurement, it is necessary to specify criteria such as the number of readings, the period of rest before the readings are taken, whether the subject should be sitting or supine, the necessity to use the same type of sphygmomanometer, the number of readings to take, whether one records the best or the average of a specified number of readings, whether readings should be recorded to the nearest mmHg or rounded up or down to the next 5 mmHg, and so on.

3. **Data from laboratory investigations and clinical tests.** Results from laboratory analysis of biological samples, or of physiological tests such as pulmonary function tests and audiometry are frequently used as part of a research project. This also requires that procedures for collection of samples, storage, and methods of analyses are consistent.

(a) *Quality control.* The laboratories should be experienced in such analyses and be participating in a quality control programme.

(b) *Calibration of equipment.* Physiological measurements should be made with calibrated equipment, using criteria which ensure that a valid test procedure is performed, and that the relevant parameters are recorded.

4. **Data obtained from medical records.** Medical records are sometimes studied in an attempt to gain clues concerning disease aetiology or associations between risk factors and disease. However, the approach is limited by the quality and completeness of the records, the people involved in keeping the records, and the purpose for which they were kept. Handwritten records may not always be legible.

5. **Data from literature review.** Research can involve trawling through the published literature for data and information from previous work on related topics. Such data may provide pointers to the present research strategy, and can help avoid unnecessary repetition of what has already been done. Published information is often in peer-reviewed journals, but some useful data may be present in books, on CD-ROM databases, or in internal reports of government departments, agencies or industry. The internet is increasingly being used as a source of data, but the quality of the data or information is very variable as there is no control over material placed on websites. Caution needs to be exercised in using data obtained this way.

6. **Qualitative research data.** Portable tape-recorders are sometimes used to record responses from participants in qualitative research. With this approach, open-ended questions are used and the responses of the participants are recorded for later analysis. The participants are free to say as little or as much as they want in response to the questions posed. Another method used to obtain data or information in qualitative research is to use focus groups.

None of these methods of obtaining data is entirely free from bias, and it is essential that such bias be minimized to ensure that the conclusions are valid.

## Methods used to reduce bias

The methods include:

- single-blind and double-blind procedures;
- training of research interviewers;
- specifying criteria for measurements;
- consistency in recording findings.

An example of a double-blind procedure is a drug trial in which neither the study participant nor the researcher knows whether the participant has been administered a drug or a placebo. With this approach of 'blinding', bias cannot be introduced, intentionally or otherwise, by either the subject or the researcher.

Laboratory animal studies are easier to control than human epidemiological studies: animals can be placed in environments where they are administered a specified treatment or placebo, whereas in human epidemiological studies, subjects may change their exposure category and this is outside the control of the researcher. Nevertheless, it is also necessary for animal studies to be subject to the rigours of standardization and consistency in data collection. These data can be similar to those outlined above (except for the use of questionnaires). Animals can be examined clinically or have biological samples collected for laboratory analysis. In addition, data can be obtained from analysis of histopathological samples after sacrifice of the animals.

## Who is involved in data collection for research projects?

- This is usually the task of one or more members of the research team working to an agreed protocol that has been approved (where relevant) by an appropriate research ethics committee, and/or an institutional review board.
- The main requirement is that those responsible for data collection should be fully familiar with the research objectives and methodology, and that they should have been trained to minimize bias in data collection.
- Where the studies involve human subjects, they should also be able to communicate clearly to the participants and explain the benefits and any inherent drawbacks to participating in the research. This aspect is often covered by a written consent form that provides an explanation and which is then signed by the participant.

## Where should data collection be done?

- Self-administered questionnaires are usually posted to the home or workplace with an addressed return envelope. The respondent can then take his/her time to complete and return the questionnaire. Groups of participants may be brought to a research office or clinic for interviewer-administered questionnaires. These may be administered singly or in groups. Where 'sensitive' questions are included, it is better for the questionnaire to be administered individually in a setting where confidentiality is assured.
- Hospital wards or clinics may be the setting for obtaining data from clinical examination or investigations.
- Occupational health studies often use workplaces for data collection.

## What steps can be taken to improve the completeness of data collection?

- The initial data set collected should be checked for completeness, and where there are items of missing data, the study subjects may have to be contacted again to obtain the missing data.
- To improve the participation rate, several strategies can be used.

  (a) A stamped return envelope may facilitate return of the information required.
  (b) Some studies pay volunteers for participation, and could be expected to have a higher participation rate, especially if payment is not provided for non-participation or incomplete participation. However, such payment may introduce bias in the recruitment of participants.

(c) A second or third reminder by letter or a follow-up phone call can be used to encourage participation. For questionnaire studies, sending out a second questionnaire in case the first has been mislaid, may increase the return rate.

Often the participation rate is dependent on the complexity of the research procedure, and the amount of data that is required.

## Further reading

Altman DG. *Practical Statistics for Medical Research.* London: Chapman & Hall, 1997.

Aw TC. Research in occupational medicine: research methodology. *Occupational Medicine* 1997; **47**: 432–434.

O'Rourke MK. Principles of epidemiology. In: JB Sullivan, GR Kreiger, (eds). *Clinical Environmental Health and Toxic Exposures* (2nd ed), Philadelphia, Lippincott Williams & Wilkins, 2001.

## Related topics of interest

Measurements, p. 68; Research process, p. 6; Research design, p. 31.

# MEASUREMENTS

*Taj Dhallu, Fang Gao Smith*

Medical research involves the measurement of biological variables such as blood pressure, plasma urea, birth weight, etc. Clearly, measurements should reflect the true, underlying value of the variable under scrutiny as closely as possible, if the research findings are to be regarded as reliable. It is therefore important to understand the factors that may affect the accuracy of measurements in research.

## Accuracy of measurements

To be accurate, one must be able to measure the quantity precisely and without bias. These concepts can be understood in the context of making several measurements of arterial blood pressure with a sphygmomanometer. (It is assumed that it is possible to measure the true arterial blood pressure accurately with this device.)

**1. *Precision.*** Precise and unbiased readings are readings that agree and are similar to the 'true' readings from an invasive arterial line. Precise but biased readings are readings that agree but differ consistently in one particular direction from the arterial line reading (*Figure 1*).

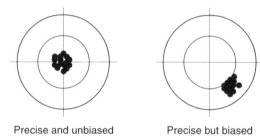

Precise and unbiased     Precise but biased

Figure 1. Precision

**2. *Bias.*** Imprecise but unbiased readings are randomly scattered around the true values from the arterial line pressure. Biased and imprecise readings are scattered but tend to differ consistently in a particular direction from the arterial line pressure (*Figure 2*).

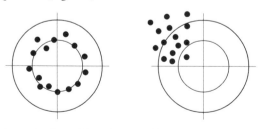

Imprecise but unbiased     Biased and imprecise

Figure 2. Bias

In summary, imprecise measurements appear random while biased measurements under- or overestimate the true value, even if precise. Generally speaking, biased data can be unbiased by comparing one value with the true value simultaneously obtained and adjusting others appropriately: imprecise data can be brought closer to the true value by taking a mean.

## Causes of measurement error

The causes of measurement error can be divided into three categories: those due to the observer, those related to the subject and those created by the measurement equipment.

**1. Observer error.** Imprecision and bias may arise when an observer repeats measurements on the same subject. This might result if, for instance, the observer is pressed for time and hurries the process of measurement.

(a) *Inter-observer inaccuracies.* These are much more common. When measurements are made by different observers on the same subject, errors commonly occur because all observers have different perceptions. In clinical trials, observers are usually 'blinded' in order to eliminate bias but this does not mean that different observers will necessarily record the same data from the same subject. For instance, the presence and severity of cyanosis will often be judged differently by different observers. Different observers may even read instrument displays differently.

(b) *Digit preference.* Digit preference is the rounding up or down of numbers. It is a common inaccuracy in the measurement of blood pressure. For example, a systolic blood pressure of 122 mmHg is often read and recorded as 120 mmHg. Different observers will round up or down differently, which can result in marked differences between the sets of observations.

(c) *Question variation.* In the case of questionnaires, responses may differ between subjects according to how the question is posed.

**2. Subject inaccuracies.**

(a) *Natural variation.* Measurements in the same subject may vary naturally. For example, three consecutive blood pressure recordings will not be exactly the same but will be grouped around some mean value. During cardiac output measurements with a pulmonary artery catheter, at least three measurements are routinely taken, which are then averaged to eliminate this type of variation. The more values that are included in the averaging process, the nearer the result is likely to be to the true value.

(b) *Unconscious bias.* Subjects may unconsciously alter measurements made upon them because of their mood. A subject's blood pressure, for instance, may increase if an attractive observer carries out the measurement.

(c) *Recall and motivation.* Information collected from questionnaires may not be reliable if the subject cannot remember or exaggerates or makes up answers to please the observer.

(d) *Compliance.* Subjects may be poorly compliant. For example, in a study to assess the effects of stopping smoking, some of the subjects may not actually stop. Some subjects may not take their prescribed medication at the appropriate times or in the correct quantity, or may not take it at all.

3. **Equipment inaccuracies.** All equipment has inherent limitations in performance. Pen recorders have inertia and frequency response limitations. Amplifiers are not necessarily linear over the full range. A full discussion is beyond the scope of this topic. Any research worker using equipment needs to have a thorough understanding of its function and limitations.

(a) *Zero errors.* Equipment such as weighing scales and electronic transducers may not be correctly zeroed, resulting in systematic errors.
(b) *Gain errors.* The calibration may not be accurate over the full range of measurements for which the equipment is used.
(c) *Precision.* The use of reagent strips, such as BM-Test to measure blood sugar, may not be sensitive enough for some studies.

## Assessment of the accuracy of measurement

There are many statistical tests to assess the accuracy of measurements. The type of test will depend upon exactly what and how something is measured. There are some standard statistical tests to quantify agreement between different measurements.

1. **Correlation coefficient.** This is used for multiple measurements on the same subject. In order to determine how well pairs of consecutive measurements on subjects agree, a scatter diagram may be drawn and the correlation coefficient can be calculated. A standard formula gives the quantity '*r*' (see 'Correlation and regression', p. 147) which is a measure of the spread of the data around a straight line on the scatter diagram. The greater the scatter between the two consecutive measurements the lower the correlation. A strong correlation between the two measurements would give a correlation coefficient near 1 whilst poor correlation would be near 0.

2. **Standard deviation (SD).** Repeated measurements on the same subject may vary but are likely to fall into a normal distribution. On the assumption that repeated measurements on the same subject are stable, i.e. that they are unlikely to change between measurements, then any variation will be due to observer imprecision. Variance can be calculated from the differences between the consecutive measurements and the standard deviation can be calculated from the variance by taking the square root. Multiplying the standard deviation by 1.96 gives a *z* value on both sides of the mean of distribution, within which 95% of the measurements will lie. The larger the standard deviation, the lower the precision.

3. **Coefficient of variation (CV).** CV is a measure of variability relative to the mean. The standard deviation is expressed as a percentage of the mean:

$$CV = \frac{SD}{Mean} \times 100\%$$

The CV is much used in laboratory medicine. It is particularly useful when comparing the variability in two groups, since simply comparing their SDs might be misleading. For example, if plasma glucose and serum sodium analyses both had an imprecision (1 SD) of 1 mmol/l, then since this was determined at a mean glucose level of 5.0 mmol/l and a mean sodium level of 150 mmol/l, the CV of glucose assays is $1.0/5.0 \times 100\% = 20\%$ but the CV of sodium assays is $1.0/150 \times 100\% = 0.7\%$. It is generally accepted that a CV of less than 5% is acceptable reproducibility.

**4. Limits of agreement.** In clinical measurement, the comparison of a new measurement technique with an established one is needed to see whether they agree sufficiently for the new to replace the old or for the two methods to be used interchangeably. A Bland–Altman plot is the appropriate analysis. It plots the 'true' value against the difference between the two methods of measurement. The 'true' value is not known, but the best estimate for it is the mean of the two measurements.

*Figure 3* shows the comparison of oxygen saturation measured by a co-oximeter ($SaO_2$) and by a pulse oximeter ($SpO_2$). A Bland–Altman plot is used to plot the mean of $SpO_2$ and $SaO_2$ against their difference. Bias is calculated as the mean of the differences between the $SaO_2$ and $SpO_2$. Positive bias indicates that the pulse oximeter underestimates the $SaO_2$, whilst negative bias indicates that the pulse oximeter overestimates the $SaO_2$. Precision is defined as the standard deviation (SD) of these differences around the mean. The limit of agreement is taken as the bias $\pm$ (1.96 $\times$ SD), between which 95% of the differences in measurements between the two observers lie. Again, the larger the standard deviation the greater is the degree of imprecision. The correlation coefficient should not be used. The limits of agreement for $SaO_2$ and $SpO_2$ ($-1.5$ and 2.3%) are small enough for us to be confident these two methods can be used interchangeably in clinical practice.

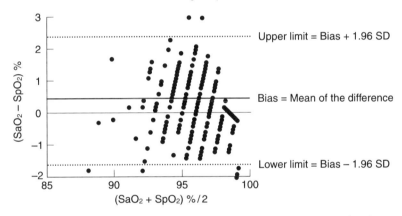

Figure 3. A Bland–Altman plot of Co-oximeter saturation and pulse oximeter saturation

# Further reading

Altman DG. *Practical Statistics for Medical Research.* London, Chapman and Hall 1991.
Bland JM, Altman DG. Statistical methods for assessing agreement between two methods of clinical measurement. *Lancet,* 1986; 1: 307–310.
Bland JM, Altman DG. Comparing methods of measurement: why plotting difference against standard method is misleading. *Lancet,* 1995; **346:** 1085–1087.
Daly LE, Bourke GJ. *Interpretation and uses of medical Statistics.* 5th edn. Oxford, Blackwell 2000.

# Related topics of interest

# DESCRIPTIVE AND INFERENTIAL STATISTICS

*Somnath Chatterjee*

Carrying out medical research involves determining values, making measurements or taking counts on a representative sample of patients, since it is impossible to study every patient within a population. The aim is to use the numerical information obtained from the sample to draw general conclusions about the whole population of similar patients. Statistical methods underpin this process of extrapolation by facilitating the manipulation, analysis and interpretation of the numerical data involved.

Statistical methods can be broadly classified into:

- Descriptive statistics
- Inferential statistics

## Descriptive statistics

*1. **Definition.*** It is the process of organizing, summarising and presenting the data obtained from the sample into a manageable size and form. No attempt is made to make inferences about the data. The end result is a concise summary of the raw data from the sample that is easier to comprehend.

*2. **Methods.*** It is firstly necessary to introduce the types of data ('Types of data' p. 74) and then go on to show how the different types of data can be summarized and presented ('Summarizing data' p. 76). It will be seen that continuous data have important distributional characteristics and in 'Measures of central tendency and dispersion' (p. 83) the methods used to define the mean and the standard deviation of the distribution will be discussed.

## Inferential statistics

Unlike the clinician, the researcher is not particularly interested in individual subjects themselves, from whom the data are collected. Usually the researcher aims to generalize or extend the findings from the sample to the entire population.

*1. **Definition.*** Inferential statistics is the process of using the data from the sample to draw conclusions or inferences about the entire population(s) of interest.

*2. **Methods.*** 'The normal distribution' (p. 89) will show how the mean and standard deviation of the sample can be used to estimate the parameters – the mean and standard deviation – of the population from which the sample was drawn. In 'Principles of statistical analysis' (p. 99) it will be shown how the means of samples vary and how this variability can be quantified in the population by confidence intervals. With this background, the principles of hypothesis testing will be discussed. Hypothesis tests use the representative samples to compare or to find associations between populations. However they do not give a simple 'yes' or 'no' answer to a research question involving comparison or association. Rather, they determine the likelihood or probability that the result is consistent with the 'null hypothesis' – that there is no difference–between the samples and therefore between the populations being studied. Subsequent topics will cover the specific statistical tests that have evolved to compare and associate sample data.

## Further reading

Clarke GM, Cooke D. *A basic course in statistics.* In: Clarke GM, Cooke D (eds), 4th edn. New York, Oxford University Press, 1998.

## Related topics of interest

Analysis of variance (AVOVA), p. 133; Chi squared and Fisher's exact test, p. 140; Measures of central tendency and dispersion, p. 83; Principles of statistical analysis – estimation and hypothesis testing, p. 99; Student's *t* test, p.110; Summarizing data, p. 76; Types of data, p. 74; Wilcoxon matched pairs signed rank sum test, p. 124.

# TYPES OF DATA

*Sukhbinder Singh*

Medical research often involves collecting information about biological characteristics, such as blood pressure or pulse rate, in a group of individuals. Many biological characteristics vary from person to person and are referred to as variables.

## Definitions

**1. Variable.** A variable may be defined as a quantity which during an investigation or experiment is assumed to vary or be capable of varying in value.

**2. Data** are the values taken by a variable.

The type of data, and the type of variable which gives rise to it, are of critical importance in determining the statistical method which can be used in the analysis of the data.

## Types of data

There are essentially two types of data: qualitative (sometimes referred to as categorical) and quantitative (also referred to as numerical) data (*Figure 1*).

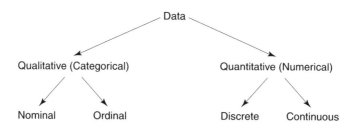

Figure 1. Types of data

**1. Qualitative data.** Qualitative or categorical data are collected when a patient is assigned to one of two or more separate categories. Words, letters or numbers may be used to label the categories. This type of data may be subdivided into nominal or ordinal data.

(a) *Nominal data.* Nominal data have categories that have no intrinsic order. Common examples include blood groups (A, B, AB or O), ethnic origin, hair colour, marital status or diagnosis. Nominal data with only two categories may be described as *dichotomous* or *binary* data. Examples include: male or female; alive or dead; smoker or non-smoker.

(b) *Ordinal data.* Ordinal data contain categories of data that have a meaningful intrinsic order. However, the differences between categories are not measurable and arithmetic processes such as adding and subtracting cannot be used. Grades of heart disease, cancer, liver cirrhosis or pre-operative fitness for surgery are examples of ordinal data. The types of labels used for the categories include: mild, moderate or severe; A, B or C; 1, 2, 3 or 4.

**2. *Quantitative data.*** Quantitative or numerical data occur when the variable can be measured and expressed numerically. Here the data values indicate both the order of the values and the distance between values. Hence arithmetic processes such as adding and subtracting can be applied to the data.

(a) *Discrete data.* Discrete data are derived from variables that can only take on certain numerical values. They arise typically from counts of events and are integers (whole numbers). Examples include the number of children in a family, the number of angina attacks per month or the number of hospital visits per year.

(b) *Continuous data.* Continuous data are where the variable can be any value within a certain range. It can be expressed to any number of decimal places if necessary. Age, height, weight, blood pressure are all continuous variables. In practice, discrete and continuous data may overlap. There are limitations in the accuracy of measurement of continuous data, e.g. height may be rounded to the nearest centimetre. Similarly, heart rate is essentially a discrete measurement but it is usually managed as a continuous measurement.

## Further reading

Daly LE. Describing data-a single variable. In: Daly LE and Bourke GJ (eds). *Interpretation and Uses of Medical Statistics.* Oxford: Blackwell Science, 2000, pp. 1–42.

## Related topics of interest

Choice of statistical tests, p. 164; Principles of statistical analysis – estimation and hypothesis testing, p. 99; Chi squared and Fisher's exact test, p. 140; Summarizing data, p. 76; Logistic regression, p. 152; Survival data, p. 155.

# SUMMARIZING DATA

*Daqing Ma, John E. Smith*

At the end of the data collection stage of a project, a set of observations will have accumulated for statistical analysis. It is difficult to comprehend the meaning or the significance of a large mass of raw data. The first step is to organize, summarize and present the data in a simple, understandable way.

## Summarizing qualitative data

**1. *Nominal data.*** The number of observations in each category (the frequency) are counted and the numbers or percentages are presented in a table or a figure. For example, the number of units of each type of blood transfused over one year on a medical ward is shown in *Table 1*.

**Table 1.** Number of units of blood group O, A, B and AB transfused over one year on Medical Ward 3

| Blood group | Number of units transfused | Percentage |
|---|---|---|
| O | 53 | 43.8 |
| A | 46 | 38.0 |
| B | 17 | 14.0 |
| AB | 5 | 4.1 |
| **Total** | **121** | **100.0** |

**2. *Ordinal data.*** *Figure 1* is a bar chart showing the Duke classifications of 157 patients treated for bowel cancer in one year. The ordinal categories are displayed on the horizontal axis and the height of each bar shows the frequency. There are spaces between the bars because the data are not continuous.

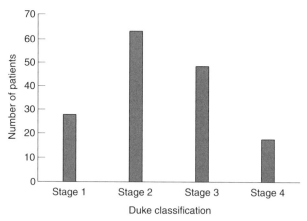

Figure 1. Number of patients with bowel cancer in Duke stages 1 to 4 treated in General Hospital 1999.

## Summarizing quantitative data

**1. Discrete data.** *Figure 2* is a bar chart showing the number of angina attacks per week in a group of 100 patients with ischaemic heart disease before and after treatment with nifedipine.

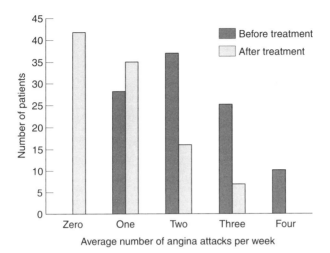

Figure 2. Average number of angina attacks per week in 100 patients before and after treatment with nifedepine.

**2. Continuous data.** Random variability has important effects on the distribution of continuous data. When measurements are taken of a continuous variable (for example blood pressure) in a sample of patients under identical conditions, the observations will vary and will be scattered over a range of values. Examination of the pattern of this data distribution is of vital importance since it will determine the type of statistical tests that can be used in the analysis of the data.

(a) *Raw data table.* *Table 2* shows the mean arterial blood pressures (MAP), taken with an automatic blood pressure monitor, of a group of 75 patients presenting

**Table 2.** Mean arterial blood pressures (mmHg) in 75 patients presenting for day case surgery

| 76 | 74 | 90 | 113 | 97 | 89 | 103 | 103 | 79 | 94 |
|-----|-----|-----|-----|-----|-----|-----|-----|-----|-----|
| 96 | 77 | 117 | 84 | 91 | 103 | 105 | 88 | 93 | 91 |
| 105 | 88 | 104 | 100 | 107 | 65 | 97 | 96 | 98 | 104 |
| 82 | 81 | 92 | 100 | 77 | 86 | 86 | 99 | 103 | 87 |
| 117 | 75 | 75 | 108 | 100 | 99 | 98 | 99 | 99 | 82 |
| 121 | 116 | 106 | 91 | 93 | 68 | 102 | 71 | 72 | 88 |
| 95 | 92 | 81 | 107 | 92 | 101 | 94 | 101 | 108 | 93 |
| 91 | 112 | 87 | 85 | 93 | | | | | |

**Table 3.** Plasma urea levels (mmol/l) in 48 patients presenting for day case surgery

| 4.3 | 3.2 | 2.7 | 5.8 | 3.1 | 4.0 | 3.7 | 4.7 |
|-----|-----|-----|-----|-----|-----|-----|-----|
| 3.0 | 3.9 | 4.1 | 3.3 | 3.7 | 4.6 | 2.8 | 2.8 |
| 5.4 | 5.3 | 3.5 | 3.3 | 2.6 | 2.9 | 6.6 | 4.3 |
| 3.2 | 3.3 | 2.4 | 7.0 | 7.2 | 3.8 | 7.5 | 4.2 |
| 3.9 | 3.9 | 3.5 | 5.2 | 3.3 | 2.8 | 3.1 | 3.9 |
| 2.4 | 4.3 | 2.7 | 3.4 | 3.1 | 2.0 | 2.6 | 2.2 |

for day-case surgery. Forty-eight of these patients also had their plasma urea levels taken (mmol/l), as shown in *Table 3*. Again, tables and figure can be used to summarize and simplify this raw data.

(b) *Frequency table.* In qualitative data the categories into which the counts are allocated are self-evident, but in continuous data, categories have to be created by grouping values of the variable. Firstly, the complete set of data is ranked and divided into 8–15 equal class intervals. For example, the MAP data can be conveniently divided into twelve 5 mmHg groups starting 65–69, 70–74, and so on, then the number of observations in each class interval are counted. This can be done easily and accurately with a computer, but without this instrument, it can be a difficult and tedious task. Perhaps the most accurate way to do it manually is to write each value on a card then deal the cards into groups corresponding to the class intervals. *Table 4* shows the tabular summary of the MAP data.

**Table 4.** Distribution of MAPs in 75 patients presenting for day case surgery

| MAP (mmHg) | Frequency |
|------------|-----------|
| 65–69 | 2 |
| 70–74 | 3 |
| 75–79 | 6 |
| 80–84 | 5 |
| 85–89 | 9 |
| 90–94 | 14 |
| 95–99 | 11 |
| 100–104 | 12 |
| 105–109 | 7 |
| 110–114 | 2 |
| 115–119 | 3 |
| 120–124 | 1 |
| **Total** | **75** |

(c) *Frequency histogram.* The commonest way to illustrate a frequency distribution is by using a histogram. The successive class intervals are plotted on the horizontal axis, then bars, with heights and areas corresponding to the frequency or the relative frequency in each interval, are constructed on the intervals. *Figure 3* shows the frequency histogram of the MAP data. In frequency histograms there are no spaces between the bars because the data are continuous. The histogram presents a picture of the distribution pattern of the MAP values. It has a single peak and a roughly symmetrical shape. The frequencies tend to be clustered around one central point and the 'tails' of the distribution, near the extremes, are of similar lengths. This type of distribution is frequently seen in medicine and suggests that the sample may come from a population with a normal distribution.

(d) *Frequency polygon.* An alternative way of presenting the data is as a frequency polygon, in which the midpoints at the top of the histogram bars are joined by straight lines (*Figure 4*). If a much larger sample was studied, the class intervals could be made much smaller, the angular polygon would tend towards a smooth frequency curve.

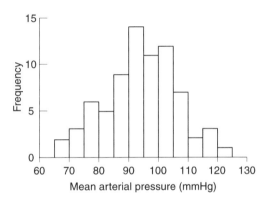

Figure 3. Frequency histogram of MAP data.

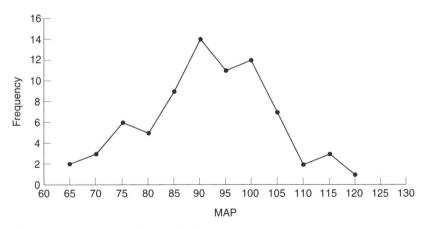

Figure 4. Frequency polygon of MAP data.

(e) *Stem-and-leaf diagram.* The stem-and-leaf diagram is a modified histogram where the bars are replaced by the numbers themselves. It has the advantage that it is simpler to draw and easier to compile from the raw data than a formal histogram. The first digit of the interval is the 'stem' and the 'leaves' are the following digits arranged in ascending order. *Figure 5* shows a stem-and-leaf plot of the MAP data.

| Interval | Stem | Leaves | | | | | | | | | | | | | |
|---|---|---|---|---|---|---|---|---|---|---|---|---|---|---|---|
| 65–69 | 6 | 5 | 8 | | | | | | | | | | | | |
| 70–74 | 7 | 1 | 2 | 4 | | | | | | | | | | | |
| 75–79 | 7 | 5 | 5 | 6 | 7 | 7 | 9 | | | | | | | | |
| 80–84 | 8 | 1 | 1 | 2 | 2 | 4 | | | | | | | | | |
| 85–89 | 8 | 5 | 6 | 6 | 7 | 7 | 8 | 8 | 8 | 9 | | | | | |
| 90–94 | 9 | 0 | 1 | 1 | 1 | 1 | 2 | 2 | 2 | 2 | 2 | 3 | 3 | 3 | 3 |
| 95–99 | 9 | 5 | 6 | 6 | 7 | 7 | 8 | 8 | 9 | 9 | 9 | 9 | | | |
| 100–104 | 10 | 0 | 0 | 0 | 1 | 1 | 2 | 3 | 3 | 3 | 3 | 4 | 4 | | |
| 105–109 | 10 | 5 | 5 | 6 | 7 | 7 | 8 | 8 | | | | | | | |
| 110–114 | 11 | 2 | 3 | | | | | | | | | | | | |
| 115–119 | 11 | 6 | 7 | 7 | | | | | | | | | | | |
| 120–124 | 12 | 1 | | | | | | | | | | | | | |

Figure 5. Stem-and-leaf diagram of MAP data.

(f) *Cumulative frequencies.* A further way of representing frequency distributions is by plotting cumulative frequencies. The cumulative frequency for a value is the number of observations in the sample with values less than or equal to that value. The relative cumulative frequency for a value is the proportion of observations in the sample with values less than or equal to that value. Hence the cumulative frequencies and relative cumulative frequencies for the MAP data are shown in *Table 5*, the cumulative frequency histogram is shown in *Figure 6* and cumulative relative frequency polygon is shown in *Figure 7*. The plots provide an easy and quick way to estimate the median and other quantiles from the distribution.

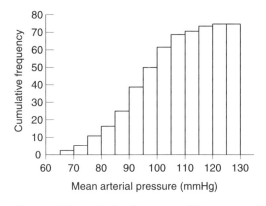

Figure 6. Cumulative frequency histogram of MAP data.

**Table 5.** Cumulative frequencies and relative cumulative frequencies of MAP data

| Class interval | Frequency | Cumulative frequency | Cumulative relative frequency % |
|---|---|---|---|
| 65–69 | 2 | 2 | 2.7 |
| 70–74 | 3 | 5 | 6.7 |
| 75–79 | 6 | 11 | 14.7 |
| 80–84 | 5 | 16 | 21.3 |
| 85–89 | 9 | 25 | 33.3 |
| 90–94 | 14 | 39 | 52 |
| 95–99 | 11 | 50 | 66.7 |
| 100–104 | 12 | 62 | 82.7 |
| 105–109 | 7 | 69 | 92 |
| 110–114 | 2 | 71 | 94.7 |
| 115–119 | 3 | 74 | 98.7 |
| 120–124 | 1 | 75 | 100 |

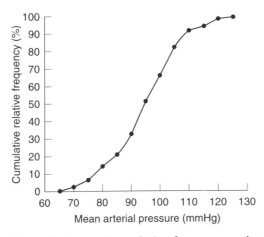

Figure 7. Cumulative relative frequency polygon of MAP data.

(g) *Skewed frequency distributions.* The histogram derived from the plasma urea data (see *Figure 8*) has a different shape than that of the BP data. It is asymmetrical and has a long right-hand tail. The distribution is skewed to the right or positively skewed. If the left tail is longer than the right the distribution is skewed to the left or negatively skewed.

## Other types of frequency distributions

Frequency distributions may assume almost any shape, but symmetrical and skewed distributions are among the most common and are the most amenable to statistical analysis. Both these distributions are unimodal, the mode being the most frequently occurring value and is represented by the peak of the frequency curve. Some distributions have two (bimodal) or more (multimodal) modes.

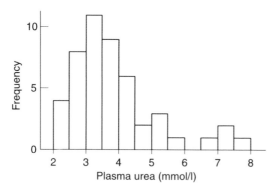

Figure 8. Frequency histogram of plasma urea data.

## Further reading

Daly LE, Bourke GJ. *Interpretation and Uses of Medical Statistics.* 5th edn, London, Blackwell Science, 2000.

## Related topic of interest

Types of data, p. 74; The normal distribution, p. 89.

# MEASURES OF CENTRAL TENDENCY AND DISPERSION

*Marcelle MacNamara, John E. Smith*

Page 77 showed the mean arterial pressure (MAP) values of 75 patients recovering from general anaesthesia and the distribution of the data was illustrated by means of a frequency histogram. The shape of the histogram emphasized two important features of the distribution. Firstly, the observations were randomly dispersed and secondly, they tended to cluster around a central point. When describing continuous data, therefore, it is essential to choose and calculate appropriate measures of both central value (central tendency) and dispersion.

## Measures of central tendency

1. ***Arithmetic mean (mean).*** The mean is the average value of the distribution. It is the sum of the observations divided by their number.

- In mathematical notation $\bar{x} = \dfrac{\sum x_1 + x_2 + x_3 \ldots \ldots x_n}{n}$

  where $\bar{x}$ is the mean, $x_1, x_2$ are the values and $n$ is the number of values. $\Sigma$ (sigma) is the summation sign. The range of values that are to be summed is often obvious, but when this is not the case, the summation sign can be used to specify it. For example $\sum_{i=1}^{n} x_i$ means the sum of all the $x_i$s from 1 to $n$, (where $x_i$ is a single observation). Hence the mean of the MAP data (p. 77) is $7032/75 = 93.76$.

- The mean is also a measure of location, it locates the point on a progressive scale around which the variables lie.

2. ***Median.*** The median is the value of the middle observation when the data are ranked in order.

- Hence, half the observations are less than or equal to it and half the observations are greater than or equal to it. For the MAP data therefore, since there are 75 observations, the median is the value of the 39th rank, 94. When there is an even number of observations, then the median is the average of the two central ranks.

- The general formula for calculating the rank of the median when there are $n$ observations is $(n+1)/2$.

- When the data have a symmetrical distribution, the values for the mean and the median will usually be fairly close. Hence, for the MAP data the mean is 93.76 mmHg and the median is 94. When data have a skewed distribution, the difference will be relatively greater. For the plasma urea data, the value of the mean is 3.84 and median is 3.5 (see *Figure 1*). The median is less affected by extreme values than is the arithmetic mean. It is particularly useful for censored data, i.e. when data above a certain value are not precisely recorded. The median is the most representative value of central tendency when no assumptions can be made about the theoretical distribution of the data, for example, data with skewed distributions.

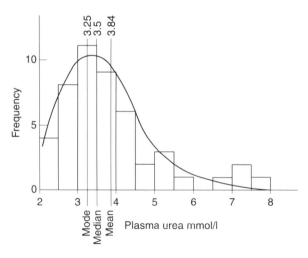

Figure 1. Mean, median and mode of plasma urea data.

**3. Mode.** The mode is the most commonly observed value. It is seldom of practical use in the statistical analysis of continuous data, indeed it can often give a misleading impression of central tendency.

**4. Geometric mean.** For skewed distributions, the geometric mean may sometimes be an alternative to the median as a measure of central tendency, as described on page 83.

## Measures of dispersion

The frequency histogram gives a useful subjective impression of the variability of a distribution but an objective, numerical description of variability is also required.

**1. Range.** The range is the difference between the highest and lowest values of the data. For the MAP data the range is 56 mmHg and for the plasma urea data it is 5.23 mg. Alternatively, the range of the MAP data may be stated as being between 68–121 mmHg and the range of the plasma urea data is between 2.0–7.5 mmol/l.

- An important disadvantage of the range as a measure of dispersion is that it depends on only the two most extreme values and therefore it is greatly affected by outliers. It does not give any information about the intermediate values in the distribution.

**2. Quantiles.** Quantiles are values that divide the distribution such that there is a given proportion of the ranked observations below the quantile.

- The median divides the distribution into two so that half the observations are less or equal to it and half are greater or equal to it.
- Quartiles divide the distribution into four equal parts.
- Centiles or percentiles are the values that divide the distribution into 100 equal parts so that a given percentage of the observations lies below a given percentile. The median is the 50th percentile, the 25th percentile is the quartile and the interquartile range lies between the first and third quartiles or the 25th and 75th percentiles.

- The effect of outliers in a distribution can be reduced by calculating the values between which, for example, 90% of the observations lie. 90% of the observations lie between the 5th and 95th percentiles. We can find out these values by ranking all the data, then calculating the rank of the 5th and 95th centile by multiplying the number of observations +1 by 0.05 and 0.95. For the plasma urea data, the 5th centile is observation $75 + 1 \times 0.05 = 3.8$, i.e. between the 3rd and the 4th observations, 2.19 and 2.34 mmol/l. The precise value can be calculated by $2.19 + 0.8(2.34 - 2.19) = 2.31$ mmol/l. Likewise the 95th centile is the observation $75 + 1 \times 0.95 = 72.2$, i.e. between the 72nd and 73rd observation. The precise value can be calculated by $6.93 + 0.2(7.05 - 6.93) = 6.95$ mmol/l. Therefore the 90% central range of the plasma urea distribution lies between 2.21 and 6.95 mmol/l.
- By specifying two values that encompass most rather than all of the data, outliers can be excluded, and many of the problems caused by specifying the gross range of the data are avoided.

**3. Box plot (box-and-whisker plot).** Several graphical methods of summarizing frequency distributions, including histograms, frequency polygons and stem-and-leaf diagrams have been described in 'Summarising data' (p. 76). The box plot, which is based on the percentile values of the distribution, is yet another way.

- In *Figure 2(a)* and *(b)*, the box represents the interquartile range, between the 25th and 75th percentiles. The median is represented by the line across the box. The ends of the 'whiskers', which extend from the box, can represent either the extreme values, as in *Figure 2(a)* and *(b)*, or the 2.5 and 97.5 percentiles, or the 10th and 90th percentiles, or any other percentile, as required. The different shapes of the MAP and plasma urea distributions can be clearly seen by comparing the two plots.

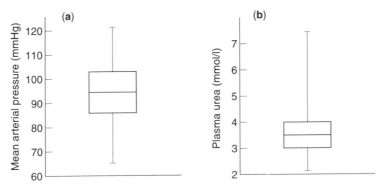

Figure 2. (a) and (b) express the percentile values of the distribution.

- A particularly useful type of box plot is shown in *Figure 3*. It identifies four outliers (represented by asterisks) at the higher end of the plasma urea distribution that are more than 1.5 times the interquartile range above the upper quartile. The interquartile range is from 2.95 to 4.3 and equals 1.35 mmol/l. 1.5 times this is 2.025. Hence 2.025 plus 4.3 equals 6.325, above which are the four observations (6.6, 7, 7.2 and 7.5). The upper whisker therefore extends to the value 5.8,

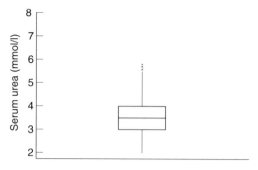

Figure 3.

which is the highest observation within this boundary. No observations are below 1.5 times the interquartile range (2.95 minus 2.025 = 0.925), so the lower whisker extends to the lowest observation (2).

**4.  Variance.** The variance and standard deviation are based on the average difference between each value in the distribution and the mean of the distribution and hence utilize all the available data.

- The difference from the mean (or the deviation from the mean) for each observation is calculated by subtracting the value of each observation from the mean $(x - \bar{x})$. If we try to average the deviations from the mean, however, we will find that the sum of the deviations is always zero, because the sum of the negative deviations is equal to the sum of the positive deviations. Therefore, each of the deviations from the mean is squared so that the values obtained are positive $(x - \bar{x})^2$. Hence adding together all the squares of the deviations from the mean is equal to $\Sigma(x - \bar{x})^2$ and is referred to as the sum of squares. The average of this is a measure of the amount of variability of the data and is termed *variance* and in a sample it is usually denoted by $s^2$.

$$\text{Variance} = s^2 = \frac{\sqrt{(x - \bar{x})^2}}{n - 1}$$

- In this equation $n - 1$ is used rather than $n$ because it can be shown mathematically that in small samples, the use of $n - 1$ gives a better estimation of the variance and standard deviation of the population from which the sample was drawn. As the sample size increases, the difference between the divisors $n$ and $n - 1$ becomes less and less significant. For example, in the MAP sample: Variance = 11033/74 = 149.1 square mmHg.

**5.  Standard deviation.** The variance is of limited value as a summary statistic because it is expressed in different units from those of the observations themselves. We wish to summarize the variability of the BP data not in square mmHg but in mmHg. Taking the square root of the variance produces the standard deviation ($s$, $sd$ or $SD$) of the sample, which has the same units as the observations and the mean. Hence:

$$s = \sqrt{\frac{\Sigma(x - \bar{x})^2}{n - 1}}$$

or rearranging:

$$s = \sqrt{\frac{\sum x^2 - \left(\sum x\right)^2 / n}{n-1}}$$

Hence for the MAP data:

$$\sum x^2 = 670354 \ \left(\sum x^2 = x_1^2 + x_2^2 + x_3^2 \text{ and so on}\right)$$

$$\sum x = 7032$$

$$\left(\sum x\right)^2 = 49449024$$

$$s = \sqrt{\frac{670354 - 49449024/75}{74}}$$

$$= 12.21 \,\text{mmHg}$$

- The standard deviation has an important role as a measure of the spread of a symmetrical distribution. When comparing two data sets, the amount of variability in the distributions can be compared by comparing their standard deviations; the greater the standard deviation the greater the variability. For symmetrical distributions, it may be expected that approximately 2/3 of the observations will lie within one standard deviation of the mean and that approximately 95% of the observations will lie within two standard deviations of the mean, as will be discussed further in 'The normal distribution' (p. 89). However, this generality does not apply to asymmetrical data as will be seen in the next section.

6. **SD and skewed data.** As discussed in 'Summarising data' (p. 76) the histogram of the plasma urea data (p. 82) shows that the distribution is asymmetrical – it has a positive skew with a long right-hand tail.

- *Figures 4(a) and (b)* compare the mean and standard deviation with the median and 90% central range as summary statistics for this data. The mean is 3.84 and the SD is 1.3. The values of two standard deviations below $(3.84 - 2 \times 1.3)$ and above $(3.84 + 2 \times 1.3)$ the mean are 1.24 and 6.44 respectively. *Figure 4(a)* shows that the lower cut-off point is well below the lowest value in the distribution, whereas the upper cut-off point is exceeded by 4 observations (5.3% of the total). Hence the mean and SD do not give a helpful summary of this distribution. The median is 3.5 and the 5th and 95th percentiles are 2.29 and 7.11 respectively. These values give a clearer picture of central tendency and where the bulk of the observations lie, and are thus more appropriate summaries for this type of data.
- An alternative approach in the analysis of positively skewed data is to transform all the observations into logarithms as these may often produce a more symmetrical distribution which can be more appropriately described by the mean and standard deviation. This technique is described in 'The normal distribution' (p. 89).

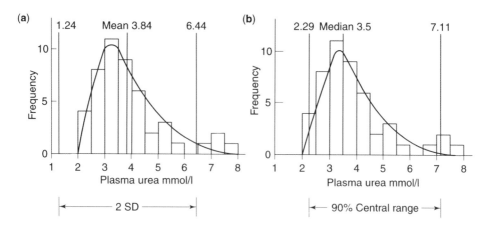

Figure 4. Plasma urea data summarized by mean ±2 SD(a) and median +90% central range (b).

## Further reading

Altman DG. *Practical Statistics for Medical Research*. London: Chapman & Hall/CRC, 1991.

## Related topics of interest

Principles of statistical analysis – estimation and hypothesis testing; p. 99; Student's *t* test, p. 110; Summarizing data, p. 76; The normal distribution, p. 89.

# THE NORMAL DISTRIBUTION

*Sukhbinder Singh, John E. Smith*

## Samples and populations

In clinical research one investigates a sample of individuals in order to use the information obtained to draw conclusions about a population of similar individuals. In statistics, the word 'population' refers to the group of individuals (which might comprise patients, objects, specimens or characteristics, etc.), in which one is interested. For example, the Mean Arterial Pressure (MAP) data tabulated in 'Summarising data' (p. 77) are from the population of 'blood pressure readings of all day-case patients presenting for general anaesthesia'.

**1. Statistical symbols.**
In this sample (p. 83) the mean and standard deviation of the variable were calculated. These are known as the statistics of the sample and are represented by the Roman letters $\bar{x}$ and $s$ respectively. The statistics are then used to make inferences about the mean and standard deviation of the population from which the sample was drawn. These values are termed the parameters of the population and are represented by Greek letters $\mu$ and $\sigma$.

**2. Inferential statistics.**
Hence, in inferential statistics, we use the sample statistics to estimate the population parameters. The word 'estimate' implies that there will always be imprecision when extrapolating sample values to the population. Probability is one of the key concepts underlying statistics and is used to quantify the uncertainties when dealing with observations, samples and populations. It is therefore necessary to review briefly the main principles of probability before going on to discuss the relationship between probability and the normal distribution.

## Probability

**1. Definition.** In statistics, the probability of an event is defined as the proportion of times the event would occur if the intervention or experiment were repeated a large number of times. It is the long-term relative frequency of the event.

**2. Properties.** Probability ($P$) is a number from 0 to 1. A probability of 1 means the event always happens and a probability of 0 means it never happens. The probability of an event not happening, therefore, is $1 - P$. Probabilities are usually expressed as decimals rather than fractions or percentages. For example, the probability of throwing a six with a dice is 0.167 (rather than 1/6 or 16.7%) and the probability of not throwing a six with a dice is $1 - 0.167 = 0.833$.

**3. Addition rule.** If two events are mutually exclusive (i.e. when one happens the other cannot happen) the probability that one or the other will happen is the sum of the individual probabilities. For example, the probability of throwing either a five or a six with a dice is $0.167 + 0.167 = 0.334$.

**4. Multiplication rule.** If two events are independent (the occurrence of one has no influence on whether the other event occurs), the probability of both events happening is the product of their probabilities. For example, the probability of throwing a six followed by another six with a dice is $0.167 \times 0.167 = 0.028$.

## The normal distribution

The histogram showing the distribution of the MAP data ('Summarising data') was based on observations from 75 patients. If it had been possible to make many thousands of such observations, the class intervals of MAP on the horizontal axis could have been made very much smaller and the frequency polygon would become a smooth curve very similar to the curve of the underlying population. This distribution is the normal or Gaussian distribution. It has a central role in statistics because of its inherent area and probability characteristics and also because the populations of many naturally occurring biological variables have normal distributions. *Figure 1* shows the normal distribution curve of the MAP of patients presenting for day-case anaesthesia. For illustrative purposes, we have assumed that the mean and SD are 93.8 and 12.2 mmHg respectively, as in the sample.

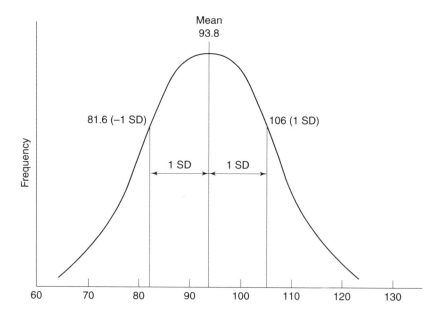

Figure 1. Normal distribution curve. Mean = 93.8, SD = 12.2.

### 1. General properties.

(a) The curve is unimodal, symmetrical and 'bell-shaped'.
(b) In theory, the tails of the distribution never touch the baseline and extend from minus infinity to plus infinity.
(c) The mean is at the midpoint of the curve, and because the distribution is unimodal and symmetrical, the median and mode are equal to the mean. The mean determines the position of the curve on the horizontal axis. If, for example, the mean of the MAP values had been greater, the curve would have been located further to the right.

(d) The standard deviation determines the spread of the curve. If, for example, the SD had been greater, the curve would have been wider and the peak relatively lower. The mean and standard deviation are the parameters of the normal distribution curve, as will be discussed later.

2. **Standard normal distribution curve.**

- Each point along the horizontal axis of a normal distribution curve can be expressed in terms of the number of standard deviations it is to the left or right of the mean. This distance (positive or negative) is known as the standard normal deviate or normal score and is indicated by z. *Figure 2* illustrates the same data as *Figure 1* but with the MAP values replaced by their standard normal deviates or z values.

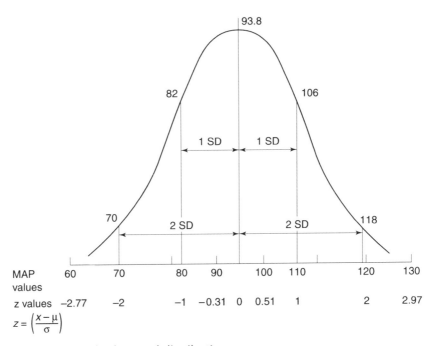

Figure 2. Standard normal distribution curve.

- The curve is now converted into the form of the standard normal distribution curve which is the theoretical model from which all normal distribution curves are derived. It has a mean ($\mu$) of zero, standard deviation ($\sigma$) of 1 and an area of 1.
- Since the area under the curve includes every possible value in the distribution, the probability of a value occurring under the curve is also 1.
- Any normal distribution can be transformed into a standard normal distribution by subtracting the mean and dividing by the standard deviation.

3. **Frequency distributions and probability distributions.**

- It is important to understand that the normal distribution curve is both a frequency distribution and a probability distribution.

- Consider the area under the standard normal distribution curve between ± one standard deviation (σ). It can be shown mathematically that this area represents 68% or a proportion of 0.68 of the total area of the curve. It can be seen intuitively, therefore, that an observation taken at random will have a chance or probability of 0.68 of being within this range and a probability of 1 − 0.68 (0.32) of being outside this range, since the probability of any value being within the curve is 1.
- Areas or proportions under a frequency distribution curve are thus equivalent to the probability of values occurring therein.

4. **Key areas and probabilities.**

- Areas or proportions can be calculated mathematically, but this is unnecessary since all the relevant areas are known and have been tabulated. Examples of the most commonly used areas are given below and in *Figure 3*.

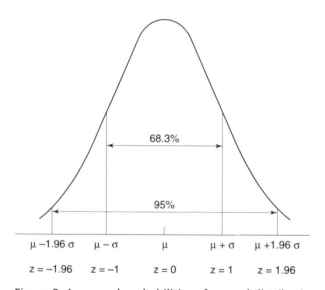

Figure 3. Areas and probabilities of normal distribution curve.

- 50% of the area lies above the mean and 50% lies below the mean. The area between +1σ and −1σ from the mean is 68% of the total area of the curve.
- The area between ±2σ from the mean is 95.4% of the total area of the curve. Hence the probability of a variable chosen at random being within this range is 0.954.
- There is a probability of 0.05 or 5% that a variable chosen at random will be outside ±1.96σ in the two tails of the distribution curve (see *Figure 3*).
- There is only a 0.0027 probability that an observation will be outside ±3σ from the mean in the tails of the distribution.

5. **One-tailed and two-tailed area tables.**

- The tails of the distribution contain the most extreme or unlikely values and they are often the areas of most interest in statistical analysis.

- There are two types of statistical tables defining areas and probabilities of the normal distribution: one-tailed area (or one-sided percentage point) and two-tailed area (two-sided percentage point) tables. The examples given above relate to two-tailed areas. They list the probability values of the standard normal distribution outside the range of a given $z$ value, where $z$ is the standard normal deviate. Hence the 5% total area outside $1.96\sigma$ from the mean comprises 2.5% in one tail and 2.5% in the other tail. One-tailed area tables list the probability values of the standard normal distribution above and below a given value of $z$, in the upper and lower tail areas.
- For both one-tailed and two-tailed areas, tables may list probabilities for given $z$ values, $(z \rightarrow P)$ or $z$ values for given probabilities $(P \rightarrow z)$.

6. **Using the normal distribution curve.** If we assume that the sample of MAP values was drawn from a population with a normal distribution of MAP values we can carry out calculations on the sample using the probability properties of the normal distribution.

*Areas in one tail – worked example 1*
(a) *Question.* What would be the chance of a pre-operative day-case patient having a MAP greater than 110 mmHg?
(b) *Calculate z value.* The mean MAP is 93.8 and the SD is 12.2 mmHg. An MAP of 110 mmHg is 16.2 mmHg above the mean. So its $z$ value, the number of standard deviations it is above the mean is $16.2/12.2 = 1.33$. It is positive, in the right side of the distribution curve.
(c) *Evaluate probability.* Table 1 is a section of the normal distribution table for areas in one tail $(z \rightarrow P)$ showing the probability of a value being above and below 1.33. The proportion of the standard normal distribution above the $z$ value of 1.33 is 0.0918 and hence the probability of a value being greater than 110 mmHg is 0.09 (9%) and the probability of a value being lower is 0.91 (91%).

**Table 1.** Extract of normal distribution table – areas in one tail $(z \rightarrow P)$

| $z$ | $P_{lower}$ | $P_{upper}$ |
| --- | --- | --- |
| 1.32 | 0.9066 | 0.0934 |
| 1.33 | 0.9082 | 0.0918 |
| 1.34 | 0.9099 | 0.0901 |

*Areas in one tail – worked example 2.*
(a) *Question.* What is the expected number of patients with a MAP between 75 and 79 mmHg in our sample of day-case patients?
(b) *Calculate z value and evaluate probability for 79 mmHg.* The $z$ value for 79 mmHg is $79 - 93.8$ (mean)$/12.2$ (SD) $= -1.21$. It is a negative value, in the left side of the distribution curve. Table 2 is a section of the normal distribution table for areas in one tail $(z \rightarrow P)$ showing the probabilities of a value being above and below 1.21. For negative values of $z$ the values of $P_{lower}$ and $P_{upper}$ are

interchanged. The proportion of the standard normal distribution below the $z$ value of −1.21 is 0.1131 and hence the probability of a value being below 79 mmHg is 0.1131.

**Table 2.** Extract of normal distribution table – areas in one tail $(z \rightarrow P)$

| $z$ | $P_{lower}$ | $P_{upper}$ |
|------|--------|--------|
| 1.20 | 0.8849 | 0.1151 |
| 1.21 | 0.8869 | 0.1131 |
| 1.22 | 0.8888 | 0.1112 |

(c) *Calculate z value and evaluate probability for 75 mmHg.* The $z$ value for 75 mmHg is 75 − 93.8(mean)/12.2(SD) = −1.54. From the normal distribution table for areas in one tail the probability of a value being below 75 mmHg is 0.0618.

(d) *Subtract probabilities.* Subtracting the probability of being below 75 mmHg from the probability of being below 79 mmHg gives the probability of values being between 75 and 79 mmHg: 0.1131 − 0.0618 = 0.0513.

(e) *Calculate number.* The expected number of (the total of 75) patients in the interval is therefore 0.0531 × 75 = 3.85. The actual number of patients in the interval was 6.

*Two-tailed areas – worked example 1*

(a) *Question.* What MAP values define the central 95% range of the MAP sample?

(b) *Find the z value.* 5% of observations will be outside the 95% range, 2.5% will be in each tail. Hence the proportion of the distribution in the two tails is 0.05. The two-tailed area normal distribution table relates the proportions and $z$ values in the tails of the distribution. We can find the $z$ value directly by using a $(P \rightarrow z)$ table or alternatively we can use the $(z \rightarrow P)$ table 'backwards.' The $z$ value corresponding to a proportion of 0.05 is shown in the section of the $(z \rightarrow P)$ table – two-tailed areas (*Table 3*). When $z$ is 1.96, a proportion of 0.05 lies outside these values.

**Table 3.** Extract of normal distribution table – two tailed areas $(z \rightarrow P)$

| $z$ | $P$ |
|------|--------|
| 1.95 | 0.0512 |
| 1.96 | 0.0500 |
| 1.97 | 0.0488 |

(c) *Calculate the range.* A $z$ value of 1.96 is 1.96 × SD = 1.96 × 12.2 = 23.9 mmHg from the mean. Hence the upper limit of the 95% central range will be 93.8 + 23.9 = 117.7 mmHg and the lower limit will be 93.8 − 23.9 = 69.9 mmHg.

## Parametric and non-parametric methods

As stated earlier, the location of a normal distribution curve can be changed by varying its mean and its spread can be changed by varying its standard deviation. The normal distribution is thus a family of distribution curves and each member of the family is defined by the specific values of its parameters, its mean and standard deviation. If we can reasonably assume (for we can never be certain) that a set of observations is from a population with a normal distribution, we can use parametric tests in the analysis of the sample. Parametric tests are based on the known parameters and the known probability properties of a distribution, in this case, the normal distribution. These tests are powerful in the sense that they utilize the actual values of the data and are therefore more likely to identify significant differences between samples of data from different populations. If no distributional assumptions can be made, samples must be analysed by non-parametric methods, which are often based on an analysis of the ranks of the data rather than the data themselves and are therefore less powerful.

## Lognormal distributions

1. *Positively skewed data.* The histogram of the plasma urea data (*Figure 4*) shows that the distribution is asymmetrical – it has a positive skew with a long right-hand tail. Clearly the raw data are not normally distributed and cannot, therefore, be analysed using parametric tests. However, transforming the data by taking the logarithm of each value may result in a distribution that is more normal.

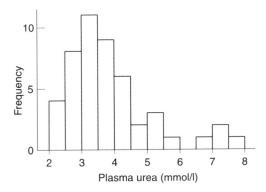

Figure 4. Histogram showing distribution of raw plasma urea data.

2. *Transformed distribution.* *Figure 5* shows the histogram of the $\log_{10}$ plasma urea data. The transformed distribution is much more symmetrical and the distribution can be tested for normality using the methods described below. If the criteria for normality are met, parametric tests can now be performed legitimately on the data.

3. *Geometric mean.* The mean of the log plasma urea data is 0.5634. If we back-transform this value (by taking the antilog) we obtain a value that is in the original units and known as the geometric mean. The geometric mean is 3.6593 mmol/l, which is very close to the value of the median (3.5 mmol/l).

4. *Definition.* If the logarithm of a set of data follows a normal distribution, the data themselves follow a lognormal distribution. Logarithmic transformation

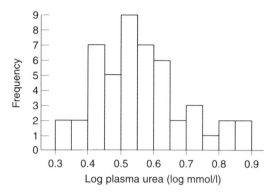

Figure 5. Histogram showing distribution of $\log_{10}$ plasma urea data.

works well for the transformation of positively skewed data because it reduces the values of the larger observations much more than it reduces the values of the smaller observations.

## Testing for normality

As discussed above, many powerful statistical tests are based on the normal distribution. Therefore, before selecting a statistical method for the analysis of a set of data, it is required that the distribution of the data is tested for its approximation to normality. There are several ways to do this:

**1. The histogram.** Simple inspection of the histogram may give a good indication of normality on some occasions. However, with small samples of, say, 15 to 20 observations, it may be very difficult to see a clear pattern.

**2. The normal plot.** The normal plot is a graphical technique that may be more reliable than inspection of the histogram.

- It is a plot of the cumulative frequency distribution for the observed data against the cumulative frequency distribution for the normal distribution.
- The data are ranked in ascending order and the expected normal score for the rank of each observation is calculated as if the data followed a standard normal distribution. There are several formulae available to facilitate this calculation.
- The numerical value of the observation is plotted along the horizontal axis and the normal score or percentage point is plotted on the vertical axis.
- If the data came from a normal distribution, the plot is very near to a straight line as shown by the normal plot of the MAP study (*Figure 6*). If the data are not normally distributed, the line is curved, as seen when the skewed data of the blood urea study are plotted (*Figure 7*).

**3. Shapiro–Wilk W test.** While inspecting the normal plot gives a subjective impression of the normality of the data, an objective measurement of the straightness or curvature of the normal plot is also available.

- The Shapiro–Wilk W test and the Shapiro–Francia W′ tests calculate the correlation coefficient as a measure of the straightness of the normal plot.

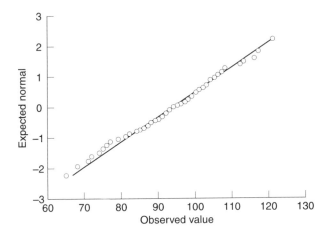

Figure 6. Normal plot of MAP data from 75 day-case patients.

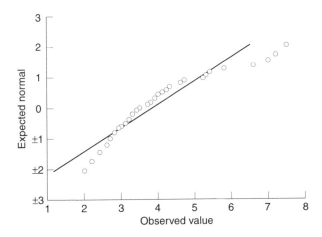

Figure 7. Normal plot of plasma urea data from 48 day-case patients.

Correlation (see 'Correlation and regression', p. 147) quantifies the straight-line association between the two continuous variables, in this case the observed data and the normal scores.

- The null hypothesis is that there is a close association, i.e. that the correlation coefficient is near to 1. Hence large values of W indicate normality and small values of W indicate non-normality. The Shapiro–Wilk table relates the probabilities associated with given W results for appropriate sample sizes. For the MAP data W is 0.989 and there is a large probability of 0.795 that the data are normal. Similarly, for the log plasma urea data (W = 0.968, P = 0.210) the null hypothesis can be accepted. However, for the plasma urea data, W is 0.885 giving a probability of <0.001 that the data are normal. Hence the null hypothesis is rejected and the data are incompatible with a normal distribution.

### 4. *Skewness and kurtosis.*

- Skewness is a measure of how symmetrically the observed values are distributed about the mean. A normal distribution has a skewness of zero.
- Kurtosis is a measure of how peaked or flat the distribution of observed values is compared to a normal distribution. A normal distribution has a kurtosis of zero.
- Problems of interpretation can arise when these two calculations reach different conclusions about the distribution. An overall measure of normality, such as W, based on the normal plot, is preferable.

## Further reading

Altman DG. Theoretical distributions. In: Altman DG (ed). *Practical Statistics for Medical Research.* London: Chapman and Hall, 1991; p. 48–73.

## Related topics of interest

Summarizing data, p. 76; Measures of central tendency and dispersion, p. 83; Principles of statistical analysis estimation and hypothesis testing, p. 99.

# PRINCIPLES OF STATISTICAL ANALYSIS – ESTIMATION AND HYPOTHESIS TESTING

*Craig Ramsay*

In most research projects the investigators wish to answer a question on a specific population within the community. For example, how many people in the UK have HIV infection or by what amount does blood pressure decrease in the over 50s when treated with different antihypertensive drugs? Although the entire population may be accessible to the investigators, in reality, financial and organizational constraints will preclude using the whole population. Therefore, investigators *sample* patients from the population of interest and then extrapolate their findings back to the entire population using statistical analysis. The one assumption underpinning this process is that the sample taken from the population is random. As a consequence of using random samples, there will always be some uncertainty about the 'real' population value and so we quantify this uncertainty by using statistical probability statements.

## Sampling and estimation

It is clear that if we take a sample of patients from the population of interest, then the true population mean ($\mu$) cannot be determined. However, we may *estimate* the population mean by taking the mean of the sample (called the sample mean, denoted by $\bar{x}$). The bigger the sample used, the closer the estimate is to the population mean (see 'Sample size and power', p. 50). In clinical practice it is rarely necessary to know the precise population mean. For example, knowing that the sensitivity of a diagnostic test was 92.13% yields the same clinical decision as knowing that the sensitivity of the test was between 91% and 93%. In addition to the population mean, it is also important to consider the variability between observations in the population. As discussed in 'Measures of central tendency and dispersion' (p. 83), the population standard deviation ($\sigma$) provides a useful measure of variability. It can be estimated using the standard deviation of the sample (called the sample standard deviation, denoted by $s$).

## Standard error of the mean (SEM)

- The sample mean is an estimate of the population mean. If we took another sample from the population, we would get a slightly different estimate of the population mean. It is, therefore, desirable to quantify the imprecision of the observed sample. To do this it is important to know that if we sample repeatedly from a normal distribution and plot the mean of each of these samples, then the corresponding distribution (known as the sampling distribution of the mean) will be normal with the mean equal to the sample mean, but the standard deviation of this distribution is given by $\frac{\sigma}{\sqrt{n}}$, where $n$ is the number of observations in the sample and $\sigma$ is the population standard deviation. The quantity $\frac{\sigma}{\sqrt{n}}$ is known as the *standard error of the mean*. We can replace $\sigma$ with the sample standard deviation, $s$.
- It is important to emphasize that if the sample is large then the sampling distribution of the mean can be assumed to be normal irrespective of the underlying

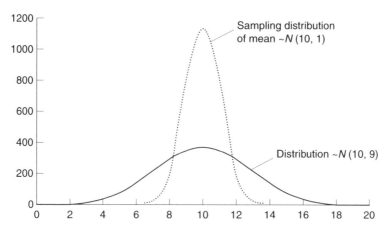

Figure 1. Normal distribution curve with mean 10 and standard deviation 3 (variance = 9), and sampling distribution curve if 2000 samples of size 9 were sampled from this normal distribution. (~N(10, 9) denotes a normal distribution curve with a mean of 10 and a variance of 9).

distribution of the sample. This feature is known as the central limit theorem. *Figure 1* illustrates a normal population with a mean of 10 and standard deviation of 3. Superimposed upon this curve is a sampling distribution of the mean if 2000 samples of size 9 were taken from this distribution – the resultant curve has the same mean of 10, but a standard deviation of $3/\sqrt{9} = 1$.

- Note that there is a difference between the standard deviation of the sample mean and the standard error of the sample mean. It is easy to muddle these up – the standard error measures the precision of the estimate, the standard deviation measures the variability of the estimate. It is the standard error of the mean that is used to quantify the imprecision of the estimate using *confidence intervals.*

## Confidence intervals

**1. Definition.** To quantify the amount by which the sample mean differs from the population mean, we find a range of values that are likely to contain the population mean. We call this range of values the *confidence interval.*

**2. Calculation.** To calculate the confidence interval (for large samples), we use a property of the normal distribution described on p. 89 – if the sampling distribution of the mean is normal, then 95% of all sample means will lie within 1.96 SEM. The 95% confidence interval is calculated as:

*sample mean* $\pm$ 1.96 $\times$ *SEM*

**3. Interpretation.** We cannot guarantee that the sample mean we observed lies within this range, there is a chance that 5% of the samples lay outwith this range. This is why we call it a 95% confidence interval. When reporting results, we write the confidence interval as (lower limit, upper limit) and say that we are 95% confident that the mean lies between these limits. We do not have to use 95% intervals. For example, we could use 99% confidence limits. This would require the SEM to be multiplied by 2.58. If we want to be more confident that the population mean is contained within the confidence interval, then the interval will get wider.

**4. An example.** Example 1 illustrates the calculation of confidence intervals. In example 1, the sampling distribution of the mean is assumed to be normally distributed because the sample size is large. Note, however, that this will not always be the case. If the sample size is small, then the assumption of normality does not hold and we would have to assume a different distribution for the mean (often assumed to be a *t*-distribution). Further discussion can be found in 'Student's *t* Test' (p. 110).

*Worked example 1. Calculating a SEM and a 95% confidence interval for large samples*
The histogram in *Figure 2* displays the distribution of phosphate levels for 105 patients with end-stage renal disease. The mean phosphate level for the 105 patients was 1.9 mmol/l and the standard deviation was 0.63. The standard error of the mean is:

$$\frac{s}{\sqrt{n}} = \frac{0.63}{\sqrt{105}} = 0.061$$

The 95% confidence interval for the mean is

$$mean \pm 1.96 \times SEM = 1.90 \pm 1.96 \times 0.061 = 1.90 \pm 0.12 = (1.78, 2.02)$$

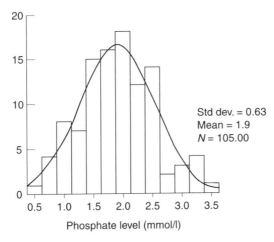

Figure 2. Distribution of phosphate levels for 105 patients with end-stage renal disease.

*Interpretation:* We are 95% confident that the mean phosphate level for patients with end-stage renal disease lies between 1.78 and 2.02 mmol/l.

## Standard error of a proportion

So far this topic has described how to calculate standard errors and confidence intervals for means. In many clinical studies, the outcome of interest is a proportion. That is, the outcome is binary (success or failure) such as alive or dead, or complication or no complication. The standard error of a proportion can be calculated easily if the sample is large.

**1. Calculation.** Assume that there were *n* individuals in the sample and *r* of these individuals had the condition of interest. The *estimated* proportion of individuals in the population with the condition is denoted by $p = r/n$. The standard error of the proportion $p$ is

$$\sqrt{\frac{p(1-p)}{n}}$$

The 95% confidence interval for the proportion is calculated the same as the mean:

$$sample\ proportion \pm 1.96 \times SE(proportion)$$

**2. An example.** For example, in a sample of 4835 births, the mode of delivery was spontaneous cephalic in 3441 cases. The estimated proportion of spontaneous cephalic deliveries in the population was $3441/4835 = 0.712$. The standard error was $\sqrt{0.712 \times (1 - 0.712)/4835} = 0.0065$ and the corresponding 95% confidence interval was $0.712 \pm 1.96 \times 0.0065 = (0.699, 0.724)$.

Note that the confidence interval of the proportion shown above is only valid if the sample is large enough for the assumption of normality of the sampling distribution of the proportion to apply. If the sample is too small, we may get impossible values (such as a negative lower bound on the confidence interval).

## Comparing the difference between two means

Although some medical research projects involve calculating estimates from a single population (as shown above), many investigations involve comparisons between subjects that have been selected from two or more populations. For example, patients with a disease compared to those without the disease or patients receiving a treatment compared to those not receiving the treatment. The investigators in such studies often want to investigate possible significant differences between the populations. It is relatively straightforward to extend the one-sample methods to compare two groups *when the samples are large*.

**1. Calculation.** In the simplest case, we have two groups of size $n_1$ and $n_2$ with sample means $\bar{x}_1$ and $\bar{x}_2$, and sample standard deviations of $s_1$ and $s_2$. We are interested in the difference between the population means and so *estimate* this difference by calculating the difference between the sample means $(\bar{x}_1 - \bar{x}_2)$. To calculate a confidence interval for the difference betwen the means we require the *standard error (se) of the difference between means*. Assuming that the samples are independent, the standard error of the difference between two means is

$$se(\bar{x}_1 - \bar{x}_2) = \sqrt{\frac{s_1^2}{n_1} + \frac{s_2^2}{n_2}}$$

and the 95% confidence interval is calculated as

$$(\bar{x}_1 - \bar{x}_2) \pm 1.96 \sqrt{\frac{s_1^2}{n_1} + \frac{s_2^2}{n_2}}$$

The 95% confidence interval for the difference gives us a range of values that we are 95% confident will contain the population difference between the means.

**2. Comparing the difference using a confidence interval.** In comparing differences between two populations, we are often interested in differences that are greater or less than zero. A confidence interval that includes zero implies that there may be no significant difference between the two populations. A confidence interval that does not include zero provides evidence that the populations are indeed different (though it is the responsibility of the researchers to decide if such differences are clinically significant).

**3. *An example and interpretation.*** Example 2 illustrates the calculation of a 95% confidence interval for a difference between means using large samples.

*Worked example 2 – Calculation of a 95% confidence interval for a difference between means using large samples.*
In a study of the birth weight of male and female babies, 1490 male babies had a mean weight of 3510 g and 1426 female babies had a mean weight of 3389 g. The standard deviations were 487 g and 465 g, respectively. The samples in this case were large enough to assume the sampling distribution of the mean difference was normal. The mean difference between the groups was $(3510 - 3389) = 121$ g. The standard error of this difference is estimated by

$$\text{se}(\bar{x}_1 - \bar{x}_2) = \sqrt{\frac{s_1^2}{n_1} + \frac{s_2^2}{n_2}} = \sqrt{\frac{487^2}{1490} + \frac{465^2}{1426}} = 17.6 \, \text{g}$$

and so the 95% confidence interval is

$$121 \pm 1.96 \times 17.6 = 121 \pm 34.5 = (86.5, \, 155.5)$$

*Interpretation:* We are 95% confident that the true difference in weight between male and female babies lies between 86.5 g and 155.5 g. In addition, the 95% confidence interval does not include zero, therefore, in this population there is evidence that the average male birth weight is heavier than the average female birth weight.

## Comparing the difference between two proportions

It is simple to extend the estimation of differences between means described above to the estimation of differences between proportions. We have two groups of size $n_1$ and $n_2$ with sample proportions $p_1$ and $p_2$. The standard error of the difference between proportions is:

$$\text{se}(p_1 - p_2) = \sqrt{\frac{p_1(1 - p_1)}{n_1} + \frac{p_2(1 - p_2)}{n_2}}$$

And given that the samples are sufficiently large, the 95% confidence interval for the difference between proportions is calculated as:

$$(p_1 - p_2) \pm 1.96 \times SE(\textit{difference between proportions})$$

## Assumptions for comparison between two groups

There were a number of assumptions made so far in this topic regarding comparing two groups:

- the groups were independent – that is, the subjects in the two groups were different;
- the difference between the groups was reflected as a difference between the population means/proportions;
- the standard deviations were the same in both groups;

- the samples were large, so the sampling distributions could be assumed to be normal.

If any of these assumptions are not valid, for example the same individuals are in the two groups (as would be the case if two biochemical tests were given to all subjects), the formulae above should not be used. Methods for investigating different types of study design are described in later topics.

## Hypothesis testing

In much of medical research, the aim of the investigation is to draw some conclusions about the differences between different populations, for example, patients with a certain condition compared to those without the condition. A *hypothesis test* allows us to measure the strength of the evidence that the groups are different. We use an 'indirect' approach to testing the hypothesis:

- Hypothesize that the groups or effects are the same (known as the *null hypothesis*).
- Find the probability (*P*-value) of observing the difference in sample means or more extreme differences if the null hypothesis were true using an appropriate statistical test.
- If the probability is low (<0.05, say), hypothesize that there is little evidence to support the null hypothesis and the groups are presumed to be different (known as the *alternative hypothesis*). If the probability is high, there is no evidence to contradict the null hypothesis and, therefore, we accept the null hypothesis.

The logic of hypothesis testing is straightforward, but there are several other factors that we must consider.

### 1. *P-values, error types and significance levels.*

- A *P*-value is a probability, and as such it introduces error into the hypothesis testing argument above. A *P*-value of 0.05 implies that 1 in 20 times we will incorrectly say there is a difference between the groups when in fact there is no difference between the groups. This is known as a *type I error*. In contrast, we can reject the alternative hypothesis when in fact it is true (*type II error*). If we decrease the risk of a type I error, we increase the chance of a type II error for a fixed sample size.
- In practice, a *P*-value less than 0.05 is usually taken to mean 'evidence of a difference'. A word of caution – there is no real difference between *P*-values of 0.06 and 0.05, so do not necessarily discard the result as non-significant. That **'P-value is significant if less than 0.05' is a guide, not a rule.** The level that we decide will provide a statistically significant result is known as the significance level. For example, if $P<0.05$ is a significant result, we state that the significance level for the test is 5%. If it was $P<0.01$, the significance level would be 1%.

### 2. *One- and two-sided tests.*

- In the format for testing hypotheses described above the anticipated direction of effect for the alternative hypothesis was not stated. The alternative hypothesis was that either group 1 was bigger than group 2 or vice versa. This is called a *two-sided* test of significance. In a *one-sided* test of significance the alternative hypothesis specifies a direction of effect. It is rare for a test to be one-sided. Only in very special cases can one be certain that the outcome will be better in one group. Of course, researchers are typically anticipating differences in many clinical trials, but the direction of the difference is not guaranteed and hence any hypothesis tests should be two-sided. So, two-sided tests should be used unless there are exceptional circumstances.

• *Figure 3* illustrates one-and two-sided tests using a standard normal distribution. If we presume a 5% significance level and a two-sided test, then we are interested in identifying the range of values in both tails of the distribution where there is, at best, a 5% chance of the values occurring. Why both tails? Because we are interested in values that are greater than the mean *and* values that are less than the mean. For example, it is equally important for us to know if drug A reduces systolic blood pressure by 5 mmHg as knowing that it increases it by 5 mmHg. Therefore *Figure 3(a)* shows the area of a standard normal curve where the probability of such a value or more extreme is 5% (0.025 + 0.025 = 0.05). In contrast, the one-sided test considers only the 5% chance of a value or more extreme in one direction of effect (as illustrated in *Figure 3(b)*). Note that if you observed a value of +1.70, then it would be statistically significant under a one-tailed test, but not with a two-tailed test (which would require a value 1.96). One-sided tests should never be used to make what should have been a non-significant two-sided test into a significant one-sided test.

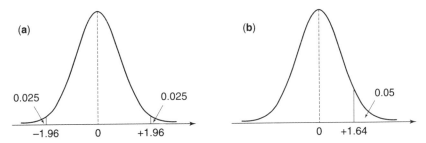

Figure 3. (a) Illustration of a 5% statistically significant area ($P < 0.05$) under a standard normal distribution for a two-sided test. (b) Illustration of a 5% statistically significant area ($P < 0.05$) under a standard normal distribution for a one-sided test.

3. **Test statistic.** Using the analogy described in the previous section, we have identified an area on the distribution that should a value occur within that area, then we believe (to 5% significance) that it provides evidence to reject the null hypothesis. We can provide statistical methods that derive where about on the distribution the sample/experiment data occurred. This method is called *calculating test statistics*. If the test statistic falls within the extremes of the distribution, the test will be statistically significant.

4. **Framework for hypothesis tests.**

• The general framework for a hypothesis test is:
   1. State the null hypothesis and the alternative hypothesis
   2. Choose the appropriate statistical test

3. Set the significance level
4. Two-sided or one-sided test?
5. Establish the critical values
6. Calculate the test statistic
7. Compare the calculated test statistic with the critical values
8. Evaluate the probability (P-value) of obtaining a result as extreme as this by chance alone, if the null hypothesis were true.

- The above framework is best illustrated by examples. We now consider two examples – the single-sample z-test (example 3) and the two-sample z-test (example 4).

*Worked example 3 – The one-sample z-test for comparing a large sample mean with a pre-specified value.*
We use the data on the 105 patients with end-stage renal disease described in example 1 to test hypotheses about the phosphate level.

1. *Question*: Was the phosphate level significantly different from 2 mmol/l in 105 patients with end-stage renal disease?
   *Null hypothesis*: Mean phosphate level $(\mu) = 2$
   *Alternative hypothesis*: Mean phosphate level not equal to 2
2., 3. and 4. There is a single sample and it is large, therefore the appropriate test of this hypothesis is *a one-sample z-test*. We shall assume *a significance level* of 5% and the test is *two-sided*.
   Using the following transformation:

   *Test statistic, z= observed sample mean – hypothesized population mean/SE (sample mean)*

   $$z = \frac{\bar{x} - \mu}{s/\sqrt{n}}$$

5. We note that $z$ is from a standard normal distribution (with mean zero and variance of one). $Z$ is known as the test statistic. We have already discussed in previous topics that if an observation lay outwith $-1.96$ and $+1.96$ on the standard normal distribution then the probability of observing such a value or more extreme value is 0.05. The values $-1.96$ and $+1.96$ are known as *the critical values*. Therefore, if the test statistic lies outwith this difference there is less than a 0.05 probability that the data arose from the null hypothesis and there would be evidence to support the alternative hypothesis.
6. *Calculate the test statistic*. In this case, the mean phosphate level was 1.90 and the standard deviation was 0.63. The z-statistic is

   $$z = \frac{1.9 - 2.0}{0.63/\sqrt{105}} = \frac{-0.1}{0.061} = -1.639$$

7. and 8. *Compare the calculated test statistic with the critical values and evaluate P-value*. This lies within $-1.96$ and $+1.96$ and so $P>0.05$. Therefore, there is no evidence that the mean phosphate level is different from 2 mmol/l.

Note that we could have answered the question using the confidence interval derived in example 1. If the 95% confidence interval included 2, then the probability of obtaining such an extreme value would have been more than 0.05 $(1-0.95)$.

As shown in example 1, the confidence interval was (1.78, 2.02) and so we could have concluded that $P > 0.05$ but in addition we also had the possible range of values that suggested that the mean phosphate level may have been less than 2. It is therefore preferable to derive the confidence interval.

*Worked example 4 – The two-sample z-test for comparing means of large samples.*
Using the data on the birth weight of male and female babies in example 2, we can test the following question:

1. *Question:* Is the birth weight of male babies different to female babies?
   *Null hypothesis:* Mean male birth weight $(\mu_1)$ = mean female birth weight $(\mu_2)$.
   *Alternative hypothesis:* Mean male birth weight is different to the mean female birth weight.
2., 3. and 4. The samples are large, therefore the appropriate test of this hypothesis is *a two-sample z-test.* We shall assume *a significance level* of 5% and the test is *two-sided.*
5. and 6. *Establish the test critical values and calculate the test statistic.* If the data are transformed as follows, the resultant z statistic will again be from a standard normal distribution: *Test statistic, z= observed sample difference in means – hypothesized population difference in means/SE (sample difference in mean)*

$$ z = \frac{(\bar{x}_1 - \bar{x}_2) - (\mu_1 - \mu_2)}{\sqrt{\dfrac{s_1^2}{n_1} + \dfrac{s_2^2}{n_2}}} $$

Under the null hypothesis the mean male birth weight, $\mu_1$, equals the mean female birth weight, $\mu_2$. This is the same as saying the difference $\mu_1 - \mu_2 = 0$. We test this hypothesis by taking the difference between the sample means.
As in example 3, the critical values for this test are $-1.96$ and $+1.96$.

In this case there were 1490 male babies with a mean birth weight of 3510 g and a standard deviation of 487 g. There were 1426 female babies with a mean weight of 3389 g and a standard deviation of 465 g. The z-statistic is:

$$ z = \frac{(3510 - 3389) - (0)}{\sqrt{\dfrac{487^2}{1490} + \dfrac{465^2}{1426}}} = \frac{121}{17.6} = 6.875 $$

7. and 8. *Compare the calculated test statistic with the critical values and evaluate P-value.* This z-statistic lies outwith $-1.96$ and $+1.96$, therefore $P < 0.05$, and so there is strong evidence that the male birth weight was greater than the female birth weight.
Again, we could have used the confidence interval for the difference to derive this result since it did not contain zero (86.5, 155.5).

Note that in the derivation of the z-statistic in the one- and two-sample z-tests the estimates are divided by the standard error of the estimates. This is the common approach for calculating test statistics. It is easy to extend the methods to investigate differences in proportions for large samples. The test statistic in this case would be the difference in proportions divided by the standard error of the difference between the proportions (formula described earlier) and again, the results would be compared to standard normal critical values.

# Hypothesis testing or confidence intervals?

There are two ways to use the standard error of an estimate (SE), either to calculate confidence intervals or for hypothesis testing. There are, however, more problems with using hypothesis tests and this has led to guidelines for publication in medical journals asking for confidence intervals in preference to, or in addition to, P-values.

### 1. The limitations of hypothesis tests are:

- The outcome of the research is determined by whether the test is significant or not, whereas, in practice, it is clinically important differences that matter.
- A difference may be statistically significant, but not practically important. If we collect a big enough sample, we can get any difference, no matter how small, to be statistically significant.
- A difference may be statistically insignificant, but there could be an important difference. A P-value greater than 0.05 does not provide evidence that there is no difference between the groups; rather it states that the difference is too small to be detected by the study.

### 2. The advantages of confidence intervals are:

- The range of plausible values for the difference are given, thereby giving readers the opportunity to judge whether the differences are clinically important.
- If the 95% confidence interval for the difference between groups does not contain zero, the result will have a less than 0.05 probability of not being significant.

# Parametric and non-parametric tests

The confidence intervals and hypothesis tests described in this topic have all assumed that the samples are large, thereby allowing the assumption of normally distributed sampling distributions to apply. Many statistical tests assume a different type of distribution (e.g. *t* distribution) because the design of the study was not as straightforward: for example, the samples are smaller. However, all of these tests are called parametric tests because they estimate effects based upon some underlying distribution. In contrast, there are some tests that do not make any assumptions of an underlying distribution and these are called non-parametric or distribution-free tests. Examples of non-parametric tests are the Mann–Whitney U test and the log-rank test for survival data. These will be described in greater detail in later topics.

# Summary

- Any research subjects are considered a *sample* from a population of possible subjects.
- We can *estimate* the population mean and standard deviation using the sample mean and sample standard deviation.
- A *confidence interval* for estimates demonstrates the range in which we believe the true population value is contained (to a given level of confidence).
- We can *test hypotheses* about these estimates by deriving probabilities from statistical tests.
- Confidence intervals should be reported in preference/addition to test statistics.

## Acknowledgement

The Health Services Research Unit is funded by the Chief Scientists Office of the Scottish Executive Health Department. The views expressed in this topic are those of the author and not necessarily those of the Department.

## Further reading

Bland M. *An Introduction to Medical Statistics.* Oxford: Oxford Medical Publication, 1995.

Gardner MJ, Altman DG. Confidence intervals rather than *P*-values: estimation rather than hypothesis testing. *British Medical Journal* 1986; **292:** 746–750.

## Related topics of interest

Choice of statistical methods, p. 164; Measures of central tendency and dispersion, p. 83; Types of data, p. 74.

# STUDENT'S *t* TEST

*Gavin D. Perkins, John E. Smith*

## Small samples and the standard error of the mean

*1. Large samples.* As discussed in the previous topic, the sampling distribution of the mean of a normal population is itself normally distributed and the standard error of the mean (the standard deviation of the sampling distribution), is calculated by: $SEM = \sigma/\sqrt{n}$ where $\sigma$ is the population standard deviation and $n$ is the number of observations in the sample. In large samples it is assumed that the sample standard deviation is a good estimate of the population standard deviation, therefore the standard error of the mean can be calculated by: $SEM = s/\sqrt{n}$ where $s$ is the standard deviation of the sample.

*2. Small samples.* In small samples, however, this assumption does not hold true because the standard deviation may vary widely from sample to sample and thus the ratio $s/\sqrt{n}$ varies widely. This increased variation is reflected in a sampling distribution of the mean known as the *t* distribution, which is more spread out and has longer tails than the normal distribution. Hence, when the sample size is small the *t* distribution is used, rather than the normal distribution, for estimation and hypothesis testing.

## The *t* distribution

*1. History.* The *t* distribution was first described by WS Gossett whilst employed at the Guinness' brewery in Dublin in 1908. The company regulations did not permit him to report his work in his own name, so he adopted the pseudonym 'Student', which is why we still refer to 'Student's *t* test'.

*2. General properties.* *t* tests are based on the *t* distribution which is a symmetrical, bell-shaped curve like the normal distribution, but having different area and probability properties. The curve is more spread out and the tails become longer as the sample size becomes smaller, reflecting the reducing precision with which $s$ estimates $\sigma$. The *t* distribution is a family of curves (*Figure 1*), which are differentiated by their degrees of freedom; the number of degrees of freedom being equivalent to sample size minus 1. With increasing sample sizes, the *t* distribution assumes the shape of the normal distribution, as the sample standard deviation becomes a better estimate of the population standard deviation.

*3. Area and probability properties.* As with the normal distribution, the area and probability properties of the *t* distribution are known and tabulated but an important difference is that these properties vary with the number of degrees of freedom. For example, the $z$ values which enclose the central 95% of the normal distribution are always 1.96, but the corresponding *t* values with a sample size of 15 (14 degrees of freedom) and 8 (7 degrees of freedom) are 2.145 and 2.365 respectively (*Figure 2*). Examples of other *t* values associated with other degrees of freedom and other two-tailed *P*-values are given in *Table 1*.

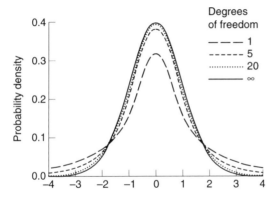

Figure 1. Graph showing normal distribution and t distribution with varying degrees of freedom. As the degrees of freedom increase the distribution becomes closer to the normal distribution.

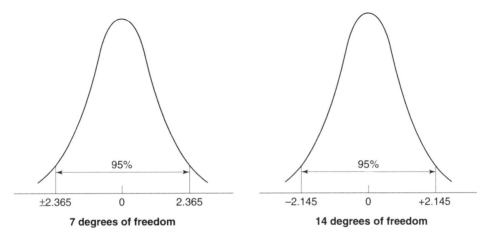

Figure 2. The t values that enclose the central 95% of the sampling distribution vary according to the number of degrees of freedom.

**Table 1.** Extract from t table (two-tailed P-values)

| Degrees of freedom $(n-1)$ | Critical value $t_c$ | | | |
|---|---|---|---|---|
| | $P=0.1$ (90% confidence) | $P=0.05$ (95% confidence) | $P=0.01$ (99% confidence) | $P=0.001$ (99.9% confidence) |
| 1 | 6.314 | 12.706 | 63.657 | 636.619 |
| 19 | 1.729 | 2.093 | 2.861 | 3.883 |
| 20 | 1.725 | 2.086 | 2.845 | 3.850 |
| 30 | 1.697 | 2.042 | 2.750 | 3.646 |
| 60 | 1.671 | 2.000 | 2.660 | 3.460 |
| 100 | 1.660 | 1.984 | 2.626 | 3.390 |
| $\infty$ | 1.645 | 1.960 | 2.576 | 3.291 |

### 4.  t or z?

In *Table 1* it can be seen that as the number of degrees of freedom increases to 100, *t* values are approaching the equivalent values found in the *z* table (e.g. when *P* is 0.05, $t = 1.984$ and $z = 1.96$) and therefore, the *t* distribution gives virtually the same results as the normal distribution. Hence, a sample size of 100 is often chosen as the cut-off point for deciding when to apply *t* or *z*. Below 100, *t* tests must be used, above 100, *z* tests could be used, though this is not essential, since *t* tests are satisfactory for the analysis of both small and large samples.

## The assumption of normality

- It should be emphasized that *z* tests, *t* tests and *F* tests (see 'Analysis of variance', p. 133) are parametric tests whose validity depends on the assumption that the sampling distribution of the mean of the population concerned is normally distributed.
- If the population itself is normally distributed, then the sampling distribution will always be normally distributed.
- In 'Principles of statistical analysis', p. 99, we also saw that if a sample is large enough, the sampling distribution of its mean can be assumed to be normally distributed even if the population from which the sample was taken has a non-normal distribution, because of the central limit theorem. It is therefore appropriate to apply parametric tests to large samples even if they have skewed distributions.
- However, this assumption cannot be made for small samples. In this context, there is no precise, clearly defined cut-off point between large and small samples, i.e. a point below which the central limit theorem can no longer assure us of a normal sampling distribution with a skewed population; much depends on factors such as the shape of the distribution, the degree of skewness, and the mean and standard deviation of the data in question. However, it may be reasonably safe to assume that many samples with more than 50 observations will have an approximately normal sampling distribution of the mean and can therefore be analysed using parametric tests.
- However, in sample sizes of less than 50, it may not be safe to assume that the sampling distribution of the population is normal. One must then use the distribution of the sample itself as a guide to the most likely distribution of the population. The histogram, the normal plot, the Shapiro–Wilk W test and the other ways to assess normality described in 'The normal distribution' (p. 89) would appear to be the right approach here. If these tests do not confirm normality, the data should be transformed and assessed again. Parametric or non-parametric tests should then be applied as appropriate.
- With very small samples, however, say, with six observations or less, it may be impossible to justify any distributional assumptions with the small amount of data available. Some statisticians therefore believe that the only valid tests are non-parametric, though other statisticians dispute this contention (see further reading).
- To summarise: Samples with more than 50 observations may usually be considered to be normally distributed. Parametric samples with less than 100 observations should usually be analysed using *t* tests rather than *z* tests.

## Confidence intervals and the *t* distribution

In small samples, from populations with normal distributions, *t* values from the *t* distribution must be used instead of *z* values from the normal distribution in calculating confidence intervals. Just as the confidence interval for a large sample is calculated as: sample mean $\pm$ $z \times$ SEM, for small samples the calculation becomes: sample mean $\pm$ $t \times$ SEM.

**1.  *Calculating a confidence interval.*** Consider a small subgroup of patients from the example given in 'Principles of statistical analysis' (p. 101) regarding phosphate levels in chronic renal failure. On this occasion the sample size was 20, but the sample mean and sample standard deviations were 1.9 mmol/l and 0.63 mmol/l as before.

(a) *The standard error of the mean.*

$$\text{SEM} = \frac{s}{\sqrt{n}} = \frac{0.63}{\sqrt{20}} = 0.14$$

(b) *The 95% confidence interval.* 95% CI for the mean is:

$$\text{Sample Mean} \pm t_c \, X \, SEM$$

where $t_c$ ($t_{critical}$) is the value which cuts off 5% of the area in the two tails of the *t* distribution. $t_c$ is derived from the *t* table for two-tailed P-values (*Table 1*) and depends on the number of degrees of freedom (number in sample $-1$). In this example the degrees of freedom are $20 - 1 = 19$ and $t_c$ is 2.093.

$$95\% \; CI = 1.9 \pm 2.093 \times 0.14 = 1.9 \pm 0.29 = (1.61, 2.19)$$

**2.  *Interpretation.*** We are 95% confident that the population mean phosphate level for patients with end-stage renal disease lies between 1.61 and 2.19 mmol/l.

**3.  *Note.*** The confidence limits here are wider than those shown in 'Principles of statistical analysis' (p. 101) (1.78, 2.02) due to the fact that there is less certainty that the standard deviation is an accurate predictor of the population value in smaller samples.

## Types of *t* tests

*t* tests, based on the *t* distribution, are used for comparing sample means of continuous quantitative data when the sample size is small (generally <100) just as *z* tests, based on the normal distribution, may be used for larger samples. *Figure 3* illustrates the types of *t* tests and outlines the situations in which they are used.

## One sample *t* test

This tests the hypothesis that the data from a single sample of patients are from a population with a known mean for the variable.

The one sample *t* test, like all other *t* tests, assumes that the sample is taken from a population with a normal sampling distribution.

*Worked example 1*
*Table 2* gives the baseline serum cholesterol data for 10 patients who are to be entered into a trial of a new cholesterol-lowering drug. The mean value of serum cholesterol in the general population is believed to be 5 mmol/l.

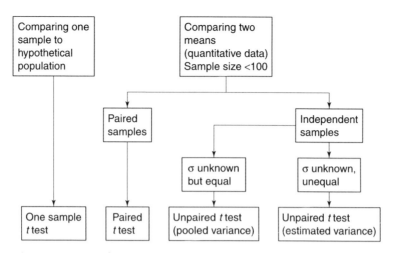

Figure 3. Types of *t* tests.

**Table 2.** Serum cholesterol levels in 10 patients

| Patient | Serum cholesterol mmol/l |
|---|---|
| 1 | 6.1 |
| 2 | 5.3 |
| 3 | 7.3 |
| 4 | 6.8 |
| 5 | 7.4 |
| 6 | 6.5 |
| 7 | 5.8 |
| 8 | 6.1 |
| 9 | 6.4 |
| 10 | 5.9 |
| **Mean** | **6.36** |
| **Std dev** | **0.66** |

*Question:* Is the level of cholesterol in the sample significantly different from the mean population value of 5 mmol/l?

*State null hypothesis (H$_0$) and the alternative hypothesis (H$_1$).*
   H$_0$: There is no difference in cholesterol levels between patients in the sample and patients in the population (i.e. the sample mean serum cholesterol = 5.0).
   H$_1$: There is a difference in cholesterol levels between patients in the sample and patients in the population (i.e. the sample mean serum cholesterol ≠ 5.0).

*Choose the appropriate statistical test.* There is one sample of patients and the population mean is known. The sample size is small, but the population from which the sample was drawn is believed to be normally distributed. The appropriate test is therefore the one-sample *t* test.

*Select the level of significance.* The *t* distribution describes the distribution of the sample means when the sample size is small as shown in *Figure 1*. The probability of another mean being from the same population as the sample mean (i.e. when the null hypothesis is true) is high when the value is close to the sample mean but lower when the value is far away from the sample mean in the extremes of the tails of the distribution. The P-value defines the cut-off points (the critical values) in the tails of the t distribution above and below which the null hypothesis is to be rejected. The nominated P-value is often taken to be 0.05, which means that the result will be considered significant if it would only occur 1 time in 20 or less when the null hypothesis is true.

*Two-sided or one-sided test?* A sample mean may be greater or smaller than the population mean so a two-sided test is required.

*Establish the critical values.* The critical values are defined by the P-value. If the P-value is 0.05 the critical values indicate the t values which separate the 95% central area of the sampling distribution of cholesterol samples (i.e. the area within which 95% of sample means will lie) from the 5% area in the tails. If the calculated t value lies between the two critical t values, the null hypothesis will be accepted. If the calculated t value lies outside the two critical t values, the null hypothesis will be rejected (*Figure 4(a)*).

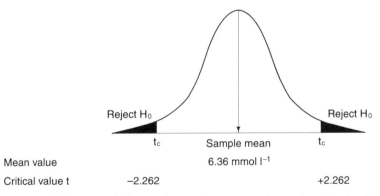

Figure 4. (a) Serum cholesterol sample mean and associated t distribution with 0.05 critical values. If the calculated value for t is less than $-2.262$ or greater than $+2.262$ it will lie outside the 95% central area of the t distribution and the null hypothesis will be rejected.

One therefore looks up the t value which corresponds to the significance level of 0.05 with $10-1=9$ degrees of freedom in the t table (*Table 3*). In this example the critical value $t_c$ is $\pm2.262$ as illustrated in *Figure 4(a)*.

**Table 3.** Extract from t table (two-tailed P-values)

| Degrees of freedom | Critical value $t_c$ | | | |
|---|---|---|---|---|
| | $P=0.1$ | $P=0.05$ | $P=0.01$ | $P=0.001$ |
| 9 | 1.833 | 2.262 | 3.250 | 4.781 |

*Calculate the test statistic.* The test statistic *t* is:

$$t = \frac{Sample\ mean - population\ mean}{Standard\ error\ of\ mean}$$

$$\frac{\bar{x} - \mu}{s/\sqrt{n}}$$

$$\frac{6.36 - 5.0}{0.66/\sqrt{10}} = \frac{1.36}{0.21} = 6.48$$

*Compare the calculated test statistic to the critical values.* The calculated *t* value lies above the critical value of $+2.262$ as illustrated in *Figure 4(b)*. The null hypothesis is therefore rejected in favour of the alternative hypothesis.

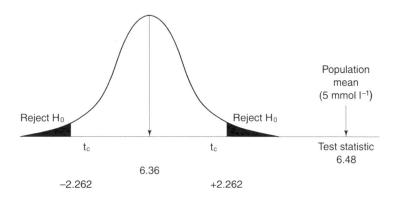

Figure 4. (b) Population serum cholesterol mean and associated test statistic *t*. The calculated value for *t* lies outside the 95% central area and the null hypothesis is rejected.

*Evaluate the probability (P-value) of obtaining a result as extreme as this by chance alone, if the null hypothesis were true.* The likelihood of obtaining a value as extreme as this by chance alone is less than 0.05 (or 1:20). From the tables (or computer program) the likelihood of obtaining this value by chance alone can be determined more accurately as $P<0.001$ (tables) or $P=0.0001$ (computer).

In this example, we conclude that the sample of cholesterol levels was significantly greater than the cholesterol levels in the general population. [6.36(0.66) versus 5. $P=0.0001$)].

*Using confidence intervals.* The difference between the sample and population mean may also be tested by calculating the 95% confidence intervals of the sample mean. If the 95% CI does not include the population mean (5), then there is less than a 5% chance that it belongs to the same population as the sample.

$$95\%\ CI = Sample\ mean \pm t_{critical} \times SEM$$

The *t* table gives the *t*-value corresponding to a tail area of 0.05 with $10-1$ degrees of freedom. Hence:

$$95\%\ CI = 6.36 \pm 2.262 \times 0.21 = (5.88,\ 6.83)$$

## Paired *t* test

**1.** *Paired data.* Paired data arise when the same individual is studied more than once (e.g. blood pressure measurements before and after treatment) or when subjects are individually matched such that only the factor under investigation is different (e.g. a matched pair case–control study).

**2.** *Indications.* The paired *t* test is used to decide whether the differences between variables measured on the same or similarly matched individuals are on average zero (in other words there is no difference between the 'before' and 'after' observations). As the data are matched there must be an equal number of observations in each sample.

**3.** *Assumption.* The paired *t* test assumes that the differences in scores between the pairs are approximately normally distributed, although the two sets of data under scrutiny do not need to be normally distributed.

*Worked example 2*
The group of 10 patients were given a course of a new cholesterol-lowering drug. The serum cholesterol level is compared after 4 weeks of treatment, and the results are shown in *Table 4*. We want to determine if the difference in cholesterol levels was due to the effect of the drug or to chance alone.

Table 4. Serum cholesterol levels before and after treatment

| Patient | Serum cholesterol before drug mmol/l | Serum cholesterol after drug mmol/l | Difference (d) |
|---|---|---|---|
| 1 | 6.1 | 6.3 | −0.2 |
| 2 | 5.3 | 4.9 | 0.4 |
| 3 | 7.3 | 6.1 | 1.2 |
| 4 | 6.8 | 5.0 | 1.8 |
| 5 | 7.4 | 7.2 | 0.2 |
| 6 | 6.5 | 4.5 | 2 |
| 7 | 5.8 | 4.8 | 1 |
| 8 | 6.1 | 5.0 | 1.1 |
| 9 | 6.4 | 4.9 | 1.5 |
| 10 | 5.9 | 5.5 | 0.4 |
| Mean | 6.36 | 5.42 | 0.94 |
| Std dev | 0.66 | 0.85 | 0.72 |

*State null hypothesis (Ho) and the alternative hypothesis (H¹).*
   $H_0$: There is no difference in serum cholesterol levels between patients treated with placebo or drug (i.e. the mean difference ($\bar{d}$) is zero).
   $H_1$: There is a difference in serum cholesterol levels in patients treated with drug compared to placebo (i.e. the mean differenced ($\bar{d}$) is not zero).

*Choose the appropriate statistical test.* In this case it is the paired *t* test, as the data are paired (two observations taken from the same patient), the differences in cholesterol levels are assumed to be normally distributed, the population variance is unknown and the sample size is small.

*Set the significance level.* A P-value of <0.05 is selected.

*Two- or one-sided test?* It is possible that the drug could have led to an increase or decrease in cholesterol, so the test needs to be two sided.

*Establish the critical values.* Calculate the degrees of freedom (number in sample −1) = 10 − 1 = 9. Determine the value of $t_c$ at the chosen level of significance (P<0.05) from the t tables (*Table 5*). These are the values between which 95% of sample means would fall if taken from the same population. If the calculated t value lies outside the critical values, the null hypothesis would be rejected in favour of the alternative hypothesis (*Figure 5(a)*).

**Table 5.** Extract from t table (two-tailed P-values)

| Degrees of freedom | Critical value $t_c$ | | | |
|---|---|---|---|---|
| | 0.1 | 0.05 | 0.01 | 0.001 |
| 9 | 1.833 | 2.262 | 3.250 | 4.781 |

As in example 1, the critical value $t_c$ is ±2.262 (*Figure 5(a)*)

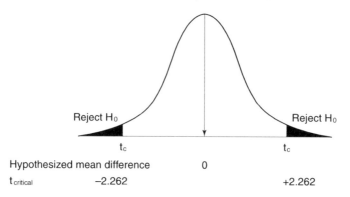

Figure 5. (a) The hypothesized mean difference between the serum cholesterol values before and after treatment (0) and associated t distribution with 0.05 critical values.

*Calculate the test statistic.* Using the following formulae:

$$t = \frac{Sample\ mean\ difference - Hypothesized\ mean\ difference}{Standard\ error\ of\ difference}$$

$$\frac{\bar{d} - 0}{s/\sqrt{n}}$$

$$\frac{0.94}{0.723/3.16} = \frac{0.94}{0.229} = 4.105$$

*Compare the calculated test statistic with the critical values.* The calculated t value (=4.105) lies above the critical value of 2.262 and therefore falls in the tail areas of the distribution where the null hypothesis is rejected (*Figure 5(b)*).

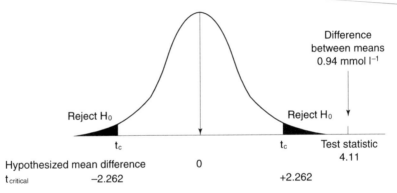

Figure 5. (b) Difference between means and associated test statistic t. The calculated value of t lies outside the 95% central area and therefore the null hypothesis is rejected.

*Evaluate the P-value.* The likelihood of obtaining a value as extreme as this by chance alone, if the null hypothesis were true, is less than 0.05 (or 1:20). From the tables (or computer program) the likelihood of obtaining this value by chance alone can be determined more accurately as $0.01 < P > 0.001$ (tables) or $P = 0.003$ (computer).

In this example, we conclude that there was a significant difference in cholesterol levels after treatment with the new drug [6.36(0.66) versus 5.42(0.85) $P = 0.003$].

*Using confidence intervals.* The differences may alternatively be presented as a 95% confidence limit.

(a) *Calculation.*

$$95\% \ CI = Mean \ difference \ (\bar{d}) \pm t_{critical} \times SE \ differences:$$

$$95\% \ CI = 0.94 \pm 2.262 \times 0.229 = 0.94 \pm 1.63 = (0.42, \ 1.46)$$

(b) *Interpretation.* As the confidence interval does not include zero it can be concluded that the new drug significantly lowered cholesterol levels.

## Unpaired or two-sample t test (equal variance assumed)

**1. Definition.** The unpaired t test is used for comparing two independent groups of observations when no suitable pairing of the observations is possible. The samples do not need to be of equal sizes. The data from most clinical trials lead to unpaired data.

**2. Assumptions.** The test requires the populations to be normally distributed with equal variance, though the test is relatively robust to deviations from these assumptions.

**3. Calculation.** The method for performing the unpaired t test is similar to that for the paired t test:

*Worked example 3*
20 symptomatic patients with asthma are entered into a placebo controlled double-blind trial of a new treatment for asthma. *Table 6* shows the results of the investigation. The investigator wants to know if the morning peak flow is significantly better

in the group of patients treated with the new drug or whether the difference is due to chance.

**Table 6.** Morning peak flow readings for patients receiving placebo and new drug

| Morning peak flow (placebo) l/min | Morning peak flow (new drug) l/min |
|---|---|
| 340 | 400 |
| 360 | 410 |
| 300 | 460 |
| 280 | 420 |
| 400 | 430 |
| 380 | 450 |
| 300 | 320 |
| 370 | 440 |
| 330 | 380 |
| | 440 |
| | 430 |
| Mean $\bar{x}_1 = 340$ | Mean $\bar{x}_2 = 416.36$ |
| $s_1 = 40.92$ | $s_2 = 39.31$ |

*State null hypothesis (H$_0$) and the alternative hypothesis (H$_1$).*

H$_0$: There is no difference in morning peak flow between patients treated with the new drug and the placebo (i.e. drug mean – placebo mean $= 0$).

H$_1$: There is a significant difference in morning peak flow between patients treated with the new drug and the placebo (i.e. drug mean – placebo mean $\neq 0$).

*Choose the appropriate statistical test.* The populations are thought to be normally distributed and the variance appears similar. The sample size is small and the data are not paired. The unpaired *t* test is therefore the appropriate test to use.

*Select the level of significance.* A P-value of $<0.05$ is selected.

*Two-sided or one-sided test?* As the drug may potentially increase or decrease the peak flow readings a two-tailed test is required.

*Establish the critical values.* Calculate the degrees of freedom: $(n_1 + n_2 - 2)$ where $n_1$ is the number of observations in the first sample and $n_2$ is the number of observations in the second sample: Df $= 9 + 11 - 2 = 18$.

Determine the critical values $t_c$ from the *t* tables (*Table 7* and *Figure 6(a)*). $t_c$ is $\pm 2.101$.

Calculate the test statistic. The test statistic *t* is

$$t = \frac{Mean\ of\ sample\ 1 - Mean\ of\ sample\ 2}{Standard\ error\ of\ difference}$$

$$= \frac{\bar{x}_1 - \bar{x}_2}{se(\bar{x}_1 - \bar{x}_2)}$$

**Table 7.** Extract from *t* table (two-tailed *P*-values)

| Degrees of freedom | Critical value $t_c$ | | | |
|---|---|---|---|---|
| | $P=0.1$ | $P=0.05$ | $P=0.01$ | $P=0.001$ |
| 18 | 1.734 | 2.101 | 2.878 | 3.922 |

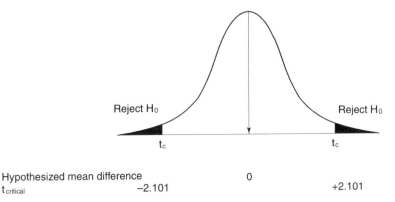

| | | | |
|---|---|---|---|
| | Reject H₀ | | Reject H₀ |
| | $t_c$ | | $t_c$ |
| Hypothesized mean difference | | 0 | |
| $t_{critical}$ | −2.101 | | +2.101 |

Figure 6. (a) The hypothesized mean difference between morning peak flows of treated group and placebo group (0) and associated *t* distribution with 0.05 critical values.

The standard error of the differences between large samples is calculated, as described in using 'Principles of statistical analysis' (p. 99):

$$se(\bar{x}_1 - \bar{x}_2) = \sqrt{\frac{s_1^2}{n_1} + \frac{s_2^2}{n_2}}$$

For small samples however, instead of using the individual variances of the two samples, the weighted average of the two sample variances, the pooled variance, $s^2_{(pooled)}$ is substituted. Hence:

$$se(\bar{x}_1 - \bar{x}_2) = \sqrt{\frac{s^2_{pooled}}{n_1} + \frac{s^2_{pooled}}{n_2}}$$

$s^2_{(pooled)}$ is calculated as follows:

$$s^2_{(pooled)} = \frac{(n_1 - 1)S_1^2 + (n_2 - 1)S_2^2}{n_1 + n_2 - 2}$$

$$= \frac{(9 - 1)(40.92)^2 + (11 - 1)(39.31)^2}{(9 + 11 - 2)} = \frac{28848.33}{18} = 1602.68$$

*t* then becomes:

$$t = \frac{\bar{x}_1 - \bar{x}_2}{\sqrt{\frac{s^2_{pooled}}{n_1} + \frac{s^2_{pooled}}{n_2}}}$$

$$= \frac{340 - 416.36}{\sqrt{\dfrac{1602.68}{9} + \dfrac{1602.68}{11}}}$$

$$= \frac{340 - 416.36}{17.99} = \frac{-76.36}{17.99} = -4.24$$

*Compare the calculated test statistic with the critical values.* The calculated $t$ value ($=-4.24$) is outside the critical value range of $-2.101$ to $+2.101$ and therefore falls in the tail areas of the distribution where the null hypothesis is rejected (*Figure 6(b)*).

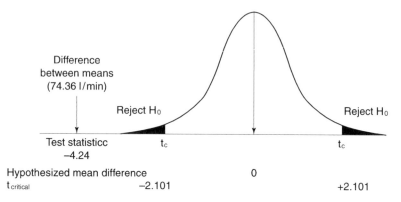

Figure 6. (b) Difference between means and associated test statistic. The calculated value of $t$ lies outside the 95% central area and therefore the null hypothesis is rejected.

*Evaluate the P-value.* The likelihood of obtaining a value as extreme as this by chance alone, if the null hypothesis were true, is less than 0.05 (or 1:20). From the tables (or computer program) the likelihood of obtaining this value by chance alone can be determined more accurately as $P<0.001$ (tables) or $P=0.0006$ (computer).

In this example one can conclude that there was a significant difference in morning peak flows between patients treated with the placebo and the new drug ($340(40.9)$ vs $416.4(39.3)$; $P<0.0006$).

*Using confidence intervals.* Alternatively the difference may be presented as a 95% confidence limit.

(a) *Calculation.*

$$95\% \; CI = \text{Mean difference} \; (\bar{x}_1 - \bar{x}_2) \pm t_{critical} \times SEM(pooled)$$

$$\text{Hence } 95\% \; CI = -76.36 \pm 2.101 \times 17.99 = (-38.6, \, -114.2)$$

(b) *Interpretation.* The confidence interval does not include zero, therefore a significant difference exists between the two treatments. It can be concluded that treatment with the new drug significantly increases peak flow (95% CI 38.6, 114.02).

## Unpaired *t* test or two-sample *t* test (unequal variance)

- When the variances of the two groups differ and transformation does not produce equal variance, the calculation of the *t* test becomes more complex.
- Instead of using the pooled variance, estimates of the individual population variances $\sigma_1^2$ and $\sigma_2^2$ are used. Test statistic:

$$t = \frac{\bar{x}_1 - \bar{x}_2}{\sqrt{(s_1^2/n_1 + s_2^2/n_2)}}$$

The test statistic may be compared to the *t* distribution with an approximation to the degrees of freedom calculated as: d.f. = the smaller of $(n_1-1)$ and $(n_2-1)$. Alternatively Welch's approximation, which is used by some computer packages (e.g. SPSS), may be used to determine the degrees of freedom.

- Alternatively a non-parametric test such as the Mann–Whitney U test may be used.

## Further Reading

Driscoll P, Lecky F. An introduction to hypothesis testing. Parametric comparison of two groups – 1. *Emergency Medical Journal* 2001; **18:**124–130.

Driscoll P, Lecky F. An introduction to hypothesis testing. Parametric comparison of two groups – 2. *Emergency Medical Journal* 2001; **18:** 214–221.

Altman DG. Comparing groups – continuous data. In: Altman DG, ed. *Practical Statistics for Medical Research.* London: Chapman and Hall. 1991; 179–228.

Daly LE, Bourke GJ. Parametric and non-parametric significance test. In: Daly LE, Bourke GJ, eds. *Interpretation and uses of Medical Statistics.* Oxford: Blackwell Science Ltd, 2000; 205–207.

Bland M. Parametric or non-parametric methods? In: Bland M, ed. An introduction to medical statistics. Oxford: Oxford University Press, 1996; 222.

## Related topics of interest

Choice of statistical methods, p. 164; Measures of central tendency and dispersion, p. 83; Principles of statistical analysis – estimation and hypothesis testing, p. 99; Types of data, p. 74.

# WILCOXON MATCHED PAIRS SIGNED RANK SUM TEST

*Gavin D. Perkins*

The Wilcoxon matched pairs signed rank sum test is the non-parametric equivalent to the paired *t* test and is used to compare data between two matched samples when the differences between the pairs are not normally distributed.

The Wilcoxon matched pairs signed rank sum tests whether two sets of related observations have the same medians. It makes no assumption about the particular shape of the distribution of the differences between the observations, but does assume that they come from a population with a symmetrical distribution. The test takes into account both the sign (positive or negative) and the magnitude of the differences between paired observations when calculating the test statistic.

Unlike the Mann–Whitney U test, transforming the data (e.g. taking the square root or logarithm) prior to analysis may alter the test result. It is therefore useful on some occasions to plot the distribution of the differences after transforming the data in order to select the more symmetrical distribution.

## Assumptions

- The paired observations are independent (i.e. the results of one pair of observations were not influenced by the results of another pair of observations).
- The differences between the pairs of observations form a symmetrical distribution (not necessarily a normal distribution).
- There are more than 6 pairs of observations.
- There are no (or few) tied values. A tie occurs when two or more subjects have the same score or value.

## Worked example

A group of students sit a multiple choice questions paper (MCQ) to test their knowledge in interpreting chest X-rays before and after a tutorial by a leading radiologist. *Table 1* shows the students' scores.

### State the null hypothesis and the alternative hypothesis.

*Null hypothesis (H₀):* There is no difference in the students' MCQ scores before and after the tutorial.

*Alternative hypothesis (H₁):* There is a significant difference in the students' MCQ scores before and after the tutorial.

### Choose the appropriate statistical test.

- The data are paired (before and after effect on the same individual), so if the differences between the two sets of observations were normally distributed then the paired *t* test could be used. However, the sample size is small and the investigator is concerned that differences may not be normally distributed.
- The data are therefore tested for normality (see 'Testing for normality' in 'The normal distribution', p. 96) and found to have a non-normal distribution.

**Table 1.** Students' MCQ scores for chest X-ray interpretation before and after a tutorial

| Student | Before | After |
|---------|--------|-------|
| 1 | 5 | 6 |
| 2 | 7 | 1 |
| 3 | 8 | 0 |
| 4 | 4 | 8 |
| 5 | 8 | 1 |
| 6 | 6 | 1 |
| 7 | 9 | 9 |
| 8 | 2 | 7 |
| 9 | 5 | 3 |
| Median | 6 | 3 |

- The differences are calculated by subtracting the score before the tutorial from the score after (*Table 2*).

**Table 2.** Differences between students' MCQ scores before and after the tutorial

| Student | Before | After | Difference |
|---------|--------|-------|------------|
| 1 | 5 | 6 | 1 |
| 2 | 7 | 1 | −6 |
| 3 | 8 | 0 | −8 |
| 4 | 4 | 8 | 4 |
| 5 | 8 | 1 | −7 |
| 6 | 6 | 1 | −5 |
| 7 | 9 | 9 | 0 |
| 8 | 2 | 7 | 5 |
| 9 | 5 | 3 | −2 |

- The differences are plotted as shown in *Figure 1*.
- The distribution of the differences around the median appears symmetrical.

Therefore, the Wilcoxon matched pairs signed rank sum test is selected.

**Set the level of significance.** Conventionally, $P < 0.05$ is considered as the level of significance.

**One- or two-sided test?** Whilst the eminent radiologist would hope that the tutorial would only improve the student's knowledge (which would need only a one-sided test), the possibility exists that it may confuse the students and worsen their MCQ score. The test is therefore two sided.

**Establish the critical values.**

- The number ($n$) of paired observations with a difference other than zero is calculated. Subject 7 had a difference in MCQ score of zero (i.e. his score was

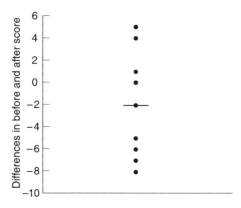

Figure 1. Plot of the differences in MCQ scores, including median value (—).

9 before and 9 after the tutorial) so his data were omitted from the calculations. Hence $n=8$.

- The critical value of the test statistic ($T$) is derived from the Wilcoxon $T$ table (two-tailed $P$-values), an extract of which is shown in *Table 3*. In this example, the critical value for $T$, corresponding to a $P$-value $<0.05$, is 3. Hence, if the test statistic is less than or equal to 3, the null hypothesis will be rejected.

**Table 3.** Extract from the Wilcoxon $T$ tables (two-tailed)

| $n$ | Two-tailed probability ($P$) | |
| | 0.05 | 0.01 |
| --- | --- | --- |
| 7 | 2 | – |
| 8 | 3 | 0 |
| 9 | 5 | 1 |

### Calculate the test statistic.

- The differences are ranked lowest to highest, ignoring the sign, in *Table 4*. The subject with zero difference is excluded from the ranking. When there are two identical values, the average of their ranks is given to each (e.g. 5 is ranked 4 and 5 so the average rank 4.5 is given).
- The ranks for all the positive differences ($\Sigma R+$) and negative differences ($\Sigma R-$) are added together

$$\Sigma R- = 6+8+7+4.5+2 = 27.5$$

$$\Sigma R+ = 1+3+4.5 = 8.5$$

- The test statistic $T$ is the smaller of $\Sigma R+$ and $\Sigma R-$. In this example $T=8.5$.

**Compare the calculated test statistic with the critical value.** The calculated value of $T$ ($=8.5$) is greater than the critical value ($=3$). It therefore falls within the area of accepting the null hypothesis.

**Table 4.** The differences in scores are ranked, excluding the sign

| Student | Before | After | Difference | Rank |
|---------|--------|-------|------------|------|
| 1 | 5 | 6 | 1 | 1 |
| 2 | 7 | 1 | −6 | 6 |
| 3 | 8 | 0 | −8 | 8 |
| 4 | 4 | 8 | 4 | 3 |
| 5 | 8 | 1 | −7 | 7 |
| 6 | 6 | 1 | −5 | 4.5 |
| 7 | 7 | 7 | 0 | |
| 8 | 2 | 7 | 5 | 4.5 |
| 9 | 5 | 3 | −2 | 2 |

*Evaluate the P-value.*

- The probability of obtaining a result this extreme, if the null hypothesis were true, is >0.05.
- The null hypothesis is therefore accepted and we conclude that there is no difference in the students' MCQ score before or after the tutorial.

## Further Reading

Bland M. Methods based on rank order. In: Bland M (ed), 2nd edn. *An Introduction to Medical Statistics.* Oxford: Oxford University Press, 1995, 205–224.

Kirkwood BR. Non-parametric methods. In: Kirkwood BR. (ed). *Essentials of Medical Statistics.* Oxford: Blackwell Science, 1988, 147–153.

Swinscow TDV. Rank score tests. In: Swinscow TDV (ed). *Statistics at Square One.* 9th edition. London: BMJ Publishing Group.1983, 92–99 (Also available on-line at http://bmj.com/collections/statsbk/10.shtml ).

## Related topics of interest

The normal distribution, p. 89; Principles of statistical analysis – estimation and hypothesis testing, p. 99.

# MANN–WHITNEY U TEST

*Gavin D. Perkins*

## Definition

The Mann–Whitney U test is the non-parametric equivalent to the unpaired *t* test. It is used to compare the medians (or location) of two unmatched samples that are not normally distributed just as the unpaired *t* test compares the means from normally distributed data. The median value (or middle value of a set of observations ranked in order) is chosen as an alternative to the mean as a measure of position as it is less sensitive to the outlying values in skewed distributions.

## Method

The Mann–Whitney U test is based on the rank order of the data rather than the actual values themselves.

- The test pools the data from the two groups and arranges them in ascending order.
- Each variable is then assigned a rank according to its position in the pooled data.
- The sum of the rank scores corresponding to the original two groups are then calculated separately. If the groups represent samples from the same population then the sum of the ranks of the two samples would be the same. If the groups represent samples from different populations then the sum of the ranks would be different. The larger the differences between the populations from which the samples were drawn, the greater the difference in the rank scores.
- The Mann–Whitney U statistic is the smaller of the sum of the ranks from the two groups and calculates the probability under the null hypothesis that the two samples are drawn from the same population.

## Assumptions

- The unpaired groups are independent (the observations in one group have no influence on the observations in the other).
- The distributions of two groups have approximately the same shape.
- There should be no tied values – a tie occurs when two or more subjects have the same score or value (although the test is reasonably robust if the number of ties is small).

## Worked example

A course of oral steroids or placebo was given in a randomized controlled trial to a group of patients with auto-immune thrombocytopenia. The platelet count after 7 days' treatment was recorded and is displayed in *Table 1*. The investigator wanted to know whether treatment with prednisolone improved the platelet count or whether the differences could be accounted for by chance.

*State the null hypothesis and the alternative hypothesis.*

*Null hypothesis* ($H_0$): there is no difference in platelet count between the group treated with steroids compared to placebo.

**Table 1.** Platelet counts in
the two groups of patients
after 7 days' treatment

| Platelet counts | |
| --- | --- |
| Placebo | Steroids |
| 49 | 90 |
| 82 | 80 |
| 54 | 100 |
| 40 | 94 |
| 20 | 84 |
| 10 | 50 |
| 60 | 12 |
| 200 | 46 |
| | 22 |
| | 12 |

*Alternative hypothesis (H₁):* there is a significant difference in platelet count between the group treated with steroids compared to placebo.

*Choose the appropriate statistical test.*

- The data are plotted to assess the shape of the underlying distributions (*Figure 1*).

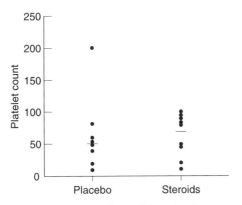

Figure 1. Distribution of data in the two groups (– is the median).

- The sample size is small and the data do not appear to be normally distributed. As the data are unpaired the Mann–Whitney U Test is the appropriate test.

*Set the level of significance.* Conventionally, $P < 0.05$ is considered as the level of significance.

*One- or two-sided test?*
As it is possible that treatment with prednisolone could either increase or decrease the platelet count, a two-sided test is required.

*Establish the critical value.*

- The critical value of the test statistic (U) is derived from the Mann–Whitney U table, an extract of which is shown in *Table 2*.

**Table 2.** Extract from Mann–Whitney U table (two-tailed)

| n1 | n2 | Two-tailed probability (P) | |
|---|---|---|---|
| | | 0.05 | 0.01 |
| 8 | 8 | 13 | 7 |
| 8 | 9 | 15 | 9 |
| 8 | 10 | **17** | 11 |
| 8 | 11 | 19 | 15 |
| 8 | 12 | 22 | 17 |

- For the sample size (8,10) at $P<0.05$, the critical value is 17. Therefore, the null hypothesis will be rejected if the calculated test statistic is less than or equal to 17.

*Calculate the test statistic.*

- The 18 observations (8 from placebo +10 from steroid group) are pooled and ranked from lowest to highest (ignoring sign if present) (*Table 3*).
- There is one tied value, so the average of the two ranks is given to each (i.e. 12 is ranked 2 and 3 and therefore the average of the ranks, 2.5, is given).
- The rank scores for each data set are summed (*Table 4*).
- The sum of the ranks for placebo $=71(R_1)$ and for steroids $=100$ ($R_2$).
- The test statistic is calculated using the formulae:

$$U_1 = R_1 - \frac{n_1(n_1 + 1)}{2}$$

$$U_2 = n_1 n_2 - U_1$$

$$U_1 = 71 - \frac{8(8 + 1)}{2} = 35$$

$$U_2 = (8)(10) - 35 = 45$$

- The test statistic U is the smaller of $U_1$ and $U_2 = 35$.

*Compare the calculated test statistic with the critical values.* The test statistic (35) is greater than the critical value (17) so the null hypothesis is accepted.

*Evaluate the P-value.*
- The chance of obtaining this result by chance alone is $>0.05$.
- The null hypothesis is accepted and the trial concludes that there was no significant difference demonstrated in platelet counts between the groups treated with steroids or placebo ($P>0.05$).

**Table 3.** The pooled and ranked data from the two groups.

| Placebo platelet count | Rank | Steroids platelet count | Rank |
|---|---|---|---|
| 10 | 1 | | |
| | | 12 | 2.5 |
| | | 12 | 2.5 |
| 20 | 4 | | |
| | | 22 | 5 |
| 40 | 6 | | |
| | | 46 | 7 |
| 49 | 8 | | |
| | | 50 | 9 |
| 54 | 10 | | |
| 60 | 11 | | |
| | | 80 | 12 |
| 82 | 13 | | |
| | | 84 | 14 |
| | | 90 | 15 |
| | | 94 | 16 |
| | | 100 | 17 |
| 200 | 18 | | |
| | Sum = 71 | | Sum = 100 |

## Mann–Whitney U test used for analysing the spread of data

When the two sample distributions are of similar shape and spread, the Mann–Whitney U test is a valid test for detecting differences in location (or medians) between two samples. However the Mann–Whitney U test can also be used to detect important differences in the shape and spread of the sample data.

- Consider the following data which represent the time delay from referral for surgery for lung cancer to the operation taking place.

  Hospital 1: Median 6.0; Interquartile range 5–70

  Hospital 2: Median 5.0; Interquartile range 2–6.75

- Applying the Mann–Whitney U test to the data gives a highly significant result ($P<0.01$).
- If the Mann–Whitney U test was regarded as simply a test of the difference in medians, then one might conclude that the difference between hospital 1 and 2 is one day's delay, which could be considered as clinically irrelevant. However, this approach would miss the important differences in the shape and spread of the data. When the data are plotted as a frequency histogram (see *Figure 2*), they clearly show that hospital 1 is providing a much poorer service, with some patients waiting up to 100 days for surgery.

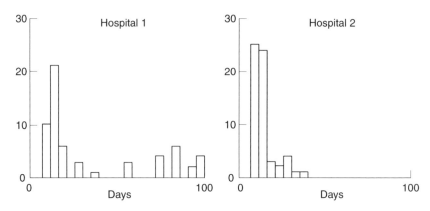

Figure 2. Time delay from referral to surgery in two hospitals.

- This example illustrates the importance of looking at the distribution of the underlying data and drawing attention to important differences in shape and spread in addition to differences in the median values.

## Nomenclature

There are two derivations of the test referred to here as the Mann–Whitney U test – one by Mann and Whitney and one by Wilcoxon. Both tests generate the same result but use slightly different methodology. To avoid confusion with the Wilcoxon matched pairs signed rank sum test for paired data (see topic on Wilcoxon matched pairs signed rank sum test, p. 124), most people refer to the Mann–Whitney U test. However, some textbooks, in order to acknowledge the contribution of Wilcoxon, may refer to the test as the Mann–Whitney–Wilcoxon test (or Wilcoxon–Mann–Whitney test).

## Further reading

Altman DG. Comparing groups – continuous data. In: Altman DG, ed. *Practical Statistics For Medical Research*. London: Chapman and Hall 1991; 194–197.

Hart A. Mann-Whitney test is not just a test of medians: differences in spread can be important. *British Medical Journal* 2001; **18**: 391–393.

# ANALYSIS OF VARIANCE (ANOVA)

Jonathan Cook

In 'Student's $t$ test' (p. 110) it was described how the $t$ test could be used to compare the means of two groups. But what if there are more than two groups? It would not be appropriate to compare every combination of the groups in pairs by using multiple $t$ tests. To do so would result in an increased risk of making a type I error. Instead an ANOVA (analysis of variance) table can be used to test for a difference in the mean outcome level between three or more groups. We define $k$ as the number of groups, $\bar{y}_i$ the mean of the $i^{th}$ group, $n_i$ as the number of observations for group $i$ and $N$ as the total number of observations. Additionally, $y_{ij}$ is the $j^{th}$ observation of the $i^{th}$ group.

## One-way ANOVA

1. **Definition.** The name Analysis of Variance (ANOVA) comes from the fact that the total variation in the data is partitioned according to the factors or categories in the model. There are a number of different ANOVA models, the simplest of which is the one-way ANOVA.

2. **Indication.** A one-way ANOVA is suitable for a continuous outcome, the same situation where we would use an independent (unpaired) $t$ test except now we have more than two groups.

3. **Hypothesis.** The hypothesis for a one-way ANOVA is:
   Question: Was there any difference in the mean level of $y$ between $k$ groups?
   Null hypothesis: Group means ($\bar{y}_i$s) are all equal.
   Alternative hypothesis: Group means are not all equal.

4. **Calculation and interpretation.** The one-way ANOVA is used to test whether or not there is a difference in the means of outcome $Y$ between $k$ groups. Under this model the total variation in the data is split into between and within groups variation. A one-way ANOVA table showing formulae is given in *Table 1*. In this table,

**Table 1.** One way ANOVA

| Source | Degrees of freedom | Sum of squares (SS) | Mean squares (MS) | F |
|---|---|---|---|---|
| Between | $k-1$ | $\sum_{ij}(\bar{y}_i-\bar{y})^2$ | $\dfrac{Between\ SS}{k-1}$ | $\dfrac{Between\ SS}{Within\ MS}$ |
| Within | $N-k$ | $\sum_{ij}(y_{ij}-\bar{y}_i)^2$ | $\dfrac{Within\ SS}{N-k}$ | |
| Total | $N-1$ | $\sum_{ij}(y_{ij}-\bar{y})^2$ | | |

$\sum_{ij}(\bar{y}_i-\bar{y})^2$ is shorthand for $\sum_{i=1}^{k}\sum_{j=1}^{n_i}(\bar{y}_i-\bar{y})^2$ and indicates double summation. It means that $(\bar{y}_i-\bar{y})^2$ is calculated and summated for each $j^{th}$ observation in each of the $k$ groups.

rows 1 and 2 correspond to the between and within variation, respectively. The between groups variation is calculated by squaring and summing the differences between the group mean $\bar{y}_i$ and the overall mean $\bar{y}$. Similarly, the within group variation is equal to squaring and summing the differences between the observed values $(y_{ij})$ and the group mean $(\bar{y}_i)$. In essence, **the one-way ANOVA estimates how much of the total variation can be attributed to differences between the groups.** The between and within sum of squares add together to give the total variation shown in the last row in *Table 1*. The mean square values are estimates of the variance and are calculated by dividing the sum of squares by the degrees of freedom. The variance ratio (F) contained in the last column is the test statistic. This value is compared with the statistical tables for a $F_{k-1, N-k}$ distribution to provide a *P*-value. When $k = 2$ this test is equivalent to the two-sample independent *t*-test.

### 5. Assumptions.

- The data for each group are assumed to be independent and normally distributed.
- The variances of the distributions are assumed equal (homoscedastic) so that the groups differ only in mean level.
- However, the test has been shown to be fairly robust to non-normal data. If the data are clearly non-normal then the non-parametric Kruskal–Wallis test can be used instead.

**6. *Multiple comparisons.*** If we have a significant result from our ANOVA we may be interested in testing which of the groups differ from each other (*post hoc* tests). Fortunately, there are a number of 'Multiple comparison tests' that allow us to do this. These tests take into account the fact that we are making multiple comparisons but tend to be over-conservative. Scheffé and least significant difference (LSD) are commonly used multiple comparison tests. Further details can be found in the further reading.

**7. *Worked example 1 – systolic blood pressure.*** We will only consider the simplest examples where the ANOVA is balanced with all treatment groups having the same number of observations. Additionally, we will only look at complete data.

A randomized controlled trial of three different drugs for hypertension has been performed. A total of 18 patients suffering from severe hypertension were randomized to receive a full course of either drug A, B or C (six patients in each treatment group). The systolic blood pressure was recorded for each patient prior to commencing treatment and upon completion of the course. The differences between these two measurements are shown in *Table 2*.

We can see that there is a difference in mean between the groups but our research question is whether this difference is due to chance (random variation) or to an actual difference in the systolic blood pressure level between the groups. Since we have more than one observation for each treatment we would call this replicate data. *Table 3* shows the ANOVA analysis.

Our main effect (drug group) is significant (*P*-value <0.05) and therefore we have evidence to reject the null hypothesis that there is no difference between the group means. The assumption of normality and homoscedasticity would need to be checked before the result is accepted.

**Table 2.** Reduction in systolic blood pressure (mmHg) by drug

|       | A     | B     | C     |
|-------|-------|-------|-------|
|       | 19.1  | 10.3  | 4.2   |
|       | 22.3  | 11.6  | 5.3   |
|       | 14.8  | 14.5  | 6.7   |
|       | 28.2  | 18.4  | 18.8  |
|       | 24.1  | 19.3  | 22.4  |
|       | 22.0  | 17.1  | 16.7  |
| Mean  | 21.75 | 15.20 | 12.35 |

**Table 3.** One-way ANOVA example

| Source  | Degrees of freedom | Sum of squares (SS) | Mean squares (MS) | F    | P-value |
|---------|--------------------|---------------------|-------------------|------|---------|
| Between | 2                  | 278.770             | 139.385           | 4.35 | 0.032   |
| Within  | 15                 | 480.510             | 32.034            |      |         |
| Total   | 17                 | 759.280             |                   |      |         |

From the group means in *Table 2* we can see that drug C must be significantly different from drug A since we have evidence that at least two of the groups differ. But, we may also be interested in the comparison of A vs B and B vs C. As described earlier, a multiple comparison test can be used to test these comparisons.

## Two-way ANOVA

1. **Definition.** The ANOVA can be extended to analyse more complicated situations than the above. The simplest extension is where we have two factors that affect the outcome. This is often called a two-way or factorial ANOVA.

2. **Worked example 2 – drug and dose.** As well as being interested in whether or not the drug has an impact on the systolic blood pressure level, we are also interested in the effect of dose level. Within the three drug groups, half the patients were randomly allocated to receive a high or low dose of the respective drug. The mean of our groups is shown in *Table 4*. A two-way ANOVA table for our trial is shown in *Table 5*.

**Table 4.** Mean reduction in systolic blood pressure by drug and dose

|      | Drug  |       |       |
|------|-------|-------|-------|
| Dose | A     | B     | C     |
| Low  | 18.73 | 12.13 | 5.40  |
| High | 24.77 | 18.27 | 19.30 |

**Table 5.** Two-way ANOVA example

| Source | Degrees of freedom | Sum of squares (SS) | Mean squares (MS) | F | P-value |
|---|---|---|---|---|---|
| Drug | 2 | 278.770 | 139.885 | 21.00 | 0.000 |
| Dose | 1 | 339.736 | 339.736 | 51.17 | 0.000 |
| Interaction | 2 | 61.108 | 30.554 | 4.60 | 0.033 |
| Residual | 12 | 79.667 | 6.639 | | |
| Total | 17 | 759.280 | | | |

**3. *Main effects and interactions.*** We now have three parts to our between treatment sum of squares: (a) a drug main effect; (b) a dose main effect and (c) an interaction. The *residual* term is equivalent to the within effect in our one-way ANOVA, i.e. it is the unexplained variance after the between treatment effects have been taken into account. This has been greatly reduced from 480.510 to 79.667 by including the dose level. Both the drug and the dose main effects are significant at the 0.1% level and hence provide very strong evidence for these effects. Notice that by taking into account the dose level, the P-value for the drug effect has been reduced. The *interaction* term tests for a non-additive relationship between the factors. Since it is significant (P-value <0.05), there is evidence that the effect of the dose level is not constant across the drugs. This can be seen in *Figure 1* where the mean reductions in systolic blood pressure are plotted. Each line corresponds to a drug group. If there was no interaction we would expect all the lines to be roughly parallel. We can clearly see that increasing the dose level has a much larger effect upon drug C than A and B.

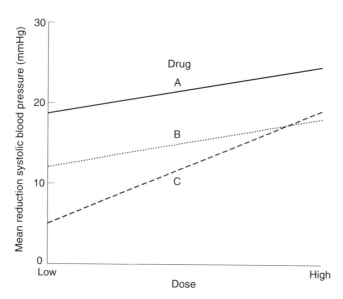

Figure 1. Mean reduction in systolic blood pressure

**4. _Number of factors._** In this example we used a $2 \times 3$ factorial ANOVA, and both of our factors were treatments, i.e. we could control the level. It is also possible to include confounders which are not controllable but known (or suspected) to be important. A common confounder is the gender of the patient. Readers are referred to further reading for a detailed discussion of ANOVA designs. Potentially, any number of factors can be included as long as there are enough observations.

**5. _Assumptions._** As for the one-way ANOVA, in producing the two-way ANOVA we are making a number of assumptions that need to be checked. The residuals, (the amount for each observation that is left unaccounted for by the main effects and interactions), are assumed to be independent and normally distributed with a constant variance.

## Repeated measures ANOVA

**1. _Definition._** The repeated measures ANOVA can be used when the groups are not independent, and can be thought of as an extension of the paired $t$-test to three or more related groups. This type of ANOVA is sometimes called a within-groups (subjects) ANOVA.

**2. _Indications._**

(a) _Different treatments to the same subject._ A situation where this type of ANOVA is used is when the $k$ treatments are given in turn to each subject. If every subject had received, in turn, a course of all three drugs in our trial, then a repeated-measures ANOVA could be used. We take repeated measures of our outcome for the same individual. The only change in circumstances between the observations from the same subject is the drug treatment.

(b) _A time course study._ Another common situation where repeated measures ANOVA are used is when we take measures for each subject at set points in time. For example we might want to measure blood pressure at 3, 4, 5 and 6 weeks of treatment.

**3. _Assumptions._** For the simplest repeated measures ANOVA:

- the data are assumed to be normally distributed;
- the subjects are assumed to be independent;
- the variance is assumed to be 'spherical'. The simplest way in which the requirements of sphericity will be satisfied is if the subjects have equal variance and the correlations for all pairs of observations are equal. This assumption is difficult to test.

**4. _Replicate and repeated measures data._** In the context of ANOVAs, the terms replicate and repeated measures data are often used:

(a) _Replicate data._ We would say that we have replicate data when we have more than one observation per treatment. As mentioned earlier, the systolic blood pressure example has replicate data since for each treatment combination (e.g. low dose of drug A), we have three observations (19.1, 22.3, 14.8). Replicate data would also occur if we chose to take replicate (multiple) measurements of a single observation, e.g. a blood pressure estimation, perhaps because we believed that our measurement of this variable may be inaccurate.

(b) *Note.* Repeated measures data are not necessarily replicate data. In this situation the factor that changes between subject measurements (usually time) is considered a treatment and therefore we have only one observation at each treatment combination.

## Kruskal–Wallis (Rank) ANOVA

**1. Definition.** Unlike the one-way ANOVA, the Kruskal–Wallis (Rank) ANOVA does not assume a distribution for the groups. Instead, it tests for a difference between the groups based upon the ranks of the observations. It is the non-parametric equivalent of the one-way ANOVA.

**2. Hypothesis.**
*Null hypothesis:* Group means are all equal.
*Alternative hypothesis:* Group means are not all equal.

**3. Calculation.** Each observation is given a rank from 1 to $N$. Let $R_i$ be the sum of the ranks for group $i$, $k$ the number of groups, $n_i$ the size of the $i^{th}$ group so that

$$\sum_{i=1}^{k} n_i = N.$$

The test statistic is:

$$\left\{ \frac{12}{N(N+1)} \sum_{i=1}^{k} \frac{R_i^2}{n_i} \right\} - 3(N+1)$$

provided there are no ties, i.e. every value is unique. The test statistic is compared to a $\chi^2$ distribution with $k-1$ degrees of freedom.

**4. Assumptions.** The groups are assumed to be independent.

**5. Worked example 3 – systolic blood pressure.** We illustrate this test using the systolic blood pressure example, ignoring the dose factor.

(a) *Rank the data as shown in* Table 6.

**Table 6.** Rank of reductions in systolic blood pressure

| Rank | Value | Drug | Rank | Value | Drug |
|------|-------|------|------|-------|------|
| 1 | 4.2 | C | 10 | 18.4 | B |
| 2 | 5.3 | C | 11 | 18.8 | C |
| 3 | 6.7 | C | 12 | 19.1 | A |
| 4 | 10.3 | B | 13 | 19.3 | B |
| 5 | 11.6 | B | 14 | 22.0 | A |
| 6 | 14.5 | B | 15 | 22.3 | A |
| 7 | 14.8 | A | 16 | 22.4 | C |
| 8 | 16.7 | C | 17 | 24.1 | A |
| 9 | 17.1 | B | 18 | 28.2 | A |

(b) *Calculate the sum of ranks.*

$$R_A = 7 + 12 + 14 + 15 + 17 + 18 = 83$$

$$R_B = 4 + 5 + 6 + 9 + 10 + 13 = 47$$

$$R_C = 1 + 2 + 3 + 8 + 11 + 16 = 41$$

(c) *Calculate the test statistic.*

$$\text{The test statistic is: } \left\{ \frac{12}{342} \times \frac{10779}{6} \right\} - 3 \times 19 = 6.035$$

(d) *Determine the P-value.* Comparing the value with $\chi^2$ distribution we see that $6.035 > \chi^2_{2,0.05} = 5.991$ and therefore we have evidence at the 5% level to reject the null hypothesis.

(e) *Note.* In this example the non-parametric (Kruskal–Wallis rank ANOVA) test resulted in the same conclusion as the one-way ANOVA. This will not always be the case. Any researcher should investigate whether the outcome is normally distributed before deciding to use the non-parametric Kruskal–Wallis test.

## Acknowledgement

The Health Services Research Unit receives core funding from the Chief Scientists Office of the Scottish Executive Health Department. The views expressed in this Topic are those of the author and not necessarily those of the Department.

## Further Reading

Armitage P, Berry G. *Statistical Methods in Medical Research.* 3rd edn. Oxford: Blackwell Scientific Publications, Oxford. 1994.

## Related topics of interest

Principles of statistical analysis – estimation and hypothesis testing, p. 99; Students' *t* test, p. 110.

# CHI SQUARED TEST AND FISHER'S EXACT TEST

*Gavin D. Perkins*

## Chi squared test

**1. Definitions.** In medical research, the most common application of the Chi squared ($\chi^2$) test is to determine if there is any association between categorical data from two or more groups.

- Categorical data are data that can be separated into distinct groups that do not have a numerical relationship or order between them.
- Examples of categorical data include eye colour, disease progression (yes/no) and blood group.

**2. Methodology.**

(a) *Make a contingency table.*
- Data are organized into a contingency table comprising rows and columns. The categories for one variable define the rows, and the categories for the other variable define the columns.
- For example, to determine if there is any association between patients taking anti-malarial drug A or B (one categorical variable) and contracting malaria (second categorical variable), data would be arranged as in *Table 1*.

**Table 1.** Infection rates according to anti-malarial medication

|  | Drug A | Drug B | Total |
|---|---|---|---|
| Malaria | 138 | 307 | 445 |
| No malaria | 12 | 43 | 55 |
| Total | 150 | 350 | 500 |

- In this format the data are referred to as a $2 \times 2$ contingency table. The $\chi^2$ test can be applied to larger tables as well. These are referred to r $\times$ c contingency tables where r = number of rows and c = number of columns.

(b) *Test the difference between observed and expected values.*
- The test compares the size of the discrepancy between the numbers observed in the rows and columns against the number that would be expected if the null hypothesis (that there are no differences between the groups) was true. If the observed and expected values are close then it would be reasonable to anticipate that the null hypothesis is true. The larger the differences between the observed and expected values, the less likely it is that the differences are due to chance alone, and the more evidence there is to reject the null hypothesis.

- The way to calculate the expected values is described below. The test statistic $\chi^2$ is calculated using the following formulae:

$$\chi^2 = \Sigma \frac{(\text{Observed} - \text{Expected value})^2}{\text{Expected value}}$$

- The test statistic is compared to the $\chi^2$ distribution. The $\chi^2$ distribution is a family of probability density curves that are defined by the number of degrees of freedom (*Figure 1*). In the *t* distribution the number of degrees of freedom depends on the sample size, but in the $\chi^2$ distribution the number of degrees of freedom depends on the number of categories and is calculated as (number of rows $-1$)$\times$(number of columns $-1$) which in this example is $(2-1)\times(2-1)=1$ degree of freedom.

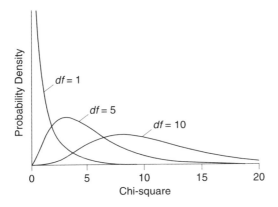

Figure 1. Probability density curves for $\chi^2$ distribution with 1, 5 and 10 degrees of freedom.

- Increasing differences between 'Observed' and 'Expected' values are reflected by an increasing value of the test statistic $\chi^2$. However, as the test statistic $\chi^2$ is a squared value it will always be positive and greater than zero irrespective of the direction of the differences between samples (i.e. greater than or less than). The right-hand tail of the $\chi^2$ distribution therefore represents the two-tailed probability that the samples were derived from the same population.
- The $\chi^2$ tests are therefore always regarded as two sided.

### 3. Assumptions.

- The sample is randomly selected from the population.
- Actual frequencies (not percentages or proportions) are entered into the contingency table.
- Observations should be independent (not paired). If the data are paired, McNemar's test should be used.
- All values must be greater than 1.
- 80% of expected values must be $>5$.

## Worked example

Two groups of patients are treated with the anti-malarial drug A or B (*Table 1*). At the end of the study 8% (12/150) of the patients treated with drug A had contracted malaria and 12.3 % (43/350) patients treated with drug B had contracted malaria. The investigator wants to establish if the difference in infection rates is due to random variation alone or if there is a real difference between the two treatments.

*State the null and alternative hypothesis.*
*Null hypothesis ($H_0$):* There is no difference in infection rates between people treated with drug A or B.

*Alternative hypothesis ($H_1$):* There is a significant difference in infection rates between people treated with drug A or B.

*Choose the appropriate statistical test.*

- The data are categorical as the patients can be divided into groups (drug A or B; infected, not infected) and there is no natural numerical relationship or order between the groups.
- It is assumed that the patients were randomly selected from the population and were randomly allocated to the two groups.
- The data are unpaired in that the study is looking at the effect of a treatment on different patients rather than a before and after effect on the same patient (which would make the data paired).

The appropriate statistical test for comparing unpaired categorical data is the $\chi^2$ test.

*Set the level of significance.* Conventionally, $P<0.05$ is considered as the level of significance.

*One- or two-sided test?* As discussed above, the $\chi^2$ test is two-sided.

*Establish the critical values.*

- The critical values are drawn from the $\chi^2$ table and are dependent on the number of degrees of freedom. This number of degrees of freedom are calculated using the formula $(r-1)\times(c-1)$, where r = number of rows, c = number of columns.
- In this example there are two rows and two columns, the degrees of freedom are therefore $(2-1)\times(2-1)=1$.
- It can be seen that in this example the critical value for $\chi^2$ corresponding to a *P*-value of 0.05 is (greater than or equal to) 3.841 (*Table 2*).

**Table 2.** Extract of $\chi^2$ table

| Degrees of freedom | Two-tailed probability | |
|---|---|---|
| | 0.05 | 0.01 |
| 1 | 3.841 | 6.635 |
| 2 | 5.991 | 9.210 |
| 3 | 7.815 | 11.345 |
| 4 | 9.488 | 13.277 |

*Calculate the test statistic.*

$$\chi^2 = \sum \frac{(\text{Observed} - \text{Expected value})^2}{\text{Expected value}}$$

- Enter actual observed values observed, 'O' (not proportions or percentages) into a 2×2 contingency table (*Table 1*).
- Calculate the expected values 'E'. The expected value is the number of patients that would have been expected to become infected in each group if the drugs had the same effect on infection rates (null hypothesis true). In this example the total proportion of patients that became infected in the trial overall was 55/500. Therefore if the null hypothesis is correct, the expected number of patients who became infected whilst on drug A is 55/500×150 = 16.5.
- The other expected frequencies may be calculated using the formula: Row total ×Column total/Overall total (*Table 3*).

**Table 3.** A table of 'observed' and 'expected' values.

|  | Drug A 'O' | Drug A 'E' | Drug B 'O' | Drug B 'E' | Total |
|---|---|---|---|---|---|
| Infected | 12 | 16.5 | 43 | 38.5 | 55 |
| Not infected | 138 | 133.5 | 307 | 311.5 | 445 |
| Total | 150 | 150 | 350 | 350 | 500 |

- Square the difference between the observed and expected value for each cell and then divide by the expected value (*Table 4*).

**Table 4.** Table containing (Observed – Expected values)$^2$/ Expected values

|  | Drug A 'O' | Drug A 'E' | Drug A $\frac{(0-E)^2}{E}$ | Drug B 'O' | Drug B 'E' | Drug B $\frac{(0-E)^2}{E}$ | Total |
|---|---|---|---|---|---|---|---|
| Infected | 12 | 16.5 | 1.22 | 43 | 38.5 | 0.53 | 55 |
| Not infected | 138 | 133.5 | 0.15 | 307 | 311.5 | 0.07 | 445 |
| Total | 150 | 150 |  | 350 | 350 |  | 500 |

- Calculate $\chi^2$ by adding these results together: $1.22 + 0.15 + 0.53 + 0.07 = 1.97$.

*Compare the calculated test statistic to the critical value.* The test statistic $\chi^2$ of 1.97 is less than the critical value of 3.841 (Table 2) and therefore falls within the area of accepting the null hypothesis.

*Evaluate P-value.* The probability of obtaining a result this extreme if the null hypothesis was true is $>0.05$.

- The null hypothesis is therefore accepted and we conclude that there is no difference in infection rates between patients treated with drug A or B (92% versus 87.7%, $\chi^2 = 1.97$, df 1, $P>0.05$).

- It is appropriate when reporting the conclusion to include percentages or proportions for each variable to aid meaningful interpretation, but as discussed above, proportions or percentages should not be included in the contingency table.

## Small sample sizes

When small sample sizes lead to expected frequencies of less than five, the assumption that the distribution of the test statistic $\chi^2$ follows the $\chi^2$ distribution may no longer be valid. In tables larger than a $2 \times 2$ table, if it is possible to merge some categories sensibly (i.e. categories can be logically combined), so that the expected number in each is greater than 5, then it may be possible to overcome this problem.

Consider the data presented in the $3 \times 2$ contingency table below (*Table 5*). It presents the results of a study that compared how frequently doctors and nurses performed cardiopulmonary resuscitation (CPR). Three cells contain an expected value of <5 which would invalidate the use of the $\chi^2$ test.

**Table 5.** Frequency of performing CPR by profession

|  | Never 'Observed' | Never 'Expected' | Infrequently 'Observed' | Infrequently 'Expected' | Frequently 'Observed' | Frequently 'Expected' |
|---|---|---|---|---|---|---|
| Doctor | 5 | 2.9 | 4 | 4.9 | 15 | 16.2 |
| Nurse | 1 | 3.1 | 6 | 5.1 | 18 | 16.8 |

However, the categories 'never' and 'infrequently' can be merged as shown in *Table 6* and then $\chi^2$ test can be performed on the resulting $2 \times 2$ table. By combining the 'never' and 'infrequently' cells, the table now fulfils the assumptions required for the $\chi^2$ test.

**Table 6.** Frequency of performing CPR by profession ('never' and 'infrequently' categories combined)

|  | Never/infrequently 'Observed' | Never/infrequently 'Expected' | Frequently 'Observed' | Frequently 'Expected' |
|---|---|---|---|---|
| Doctor | 9 | 7.8 | 15 | 16.2 |
| Nurse | 7 | 8.2 | 18 | 16.8 |

In this example it is reasonable to merge the 'never' and 'infrequently' categories as a sensible conclusion could be drawn from the new $2 \times 2$ table. This is usually possible when the categories themselves form an ordered sequence. In contrast, merging unrelated categories for example two of the four groups of the ABO blood group system, would not seem logical and should be avoided.

An alternative to merging categories is to consider analysing the data using Fisher's exact test which is described below.

## Yates continuity correction

1. **Indication.** Yates continuity correction is recommended (see further reading) when the results in a $2 \times 2$ contingency table (never for tables larger than this) total less than 100 or when any cell contains a value less than 10.

2. **The function of Yates continuity correction.** The $\chi^2$ distribution is a continuous distribution, but the observed values that are used to calculate the test statistic are discrete as they can only be whole numbers. This discrepancy may lead to the false rejection of the null hypothesis (type I error) when the number of observations are small in $2 \times 2$ tables. Yates continuity correction compensates for this problem by reducing the value of the test statistic and hence the probability that the null hypothesis will be rejected.

3. **Calculation.** The Yates continuity correction changes the $\chi^2$ formula to:

$$\chi^2 = \Sigma\left((I(O - E)I - 0.5)^2 / E\right)$$

where 'I' the vertical lines means take the absolute value of the differences between 'O' and 'E' (in other words ignore the sign).

## Other uses of chi squared test

- The chi squared ($\chi^2$) test may be used to compare an observed distribution with a theoretical distribution.
- An extension of the chi squared ($\chi^2$) test is the $\chi^2$ test for trend and may be used to compare categorical variables that have an ordering. This test takes account of the ordering to increase the statistical power of the analysis.
- A description of how to perform these tests may be found in the texts detailed in the further reading section.

## Fisher's exact test

1. **Indication.** Consider Fisher's Exact Test if:

- Total number of observations in table are less than 20.
- Total number of observations lies between 20–40 and the smallest expected (not observed) value is less than 5.

2. **The function of Fisher's exact test.** Fisher's exact test determines all the possible combinations for the observed values in the two by two table. It then compares this to the values actually observed and determines the exact probability of obtaining that result if the null hypothesis was true.

3. **Calculation.** Fisher's exact test is usually performed only on a $2 \times 2$ table, although it is now possible with some computer packages to perform the test on a table of any size.

- The main limiting factor then becomes the time it can take the computer to complete the calculation. For larger tables an alternative is to use the 'Monte Carlo' option instead, which will give a very good approximation to the exact calculation using simulation.

## Further reading

Altman DG. Comparing groups – categorical data. In: Altman DG, ed. *Practical Statistics For Medical Research*. London: Chapman and Hall; 1991; 229–276.

Swinscow TDV. The $\chi^2$ tests. In: Swinscow TDV.(ed) 9th Edition. *Statistics at Square One*. London, BMJ Publishing Group. 1983: 68–85.

## Related topics of interest

# CORRELATION AND REGRESSION

*Daqing Ma, Fang Gao Smith*

Correlation and regression are the two methods commonly used to assess the relationship between two continuous variables within a group of subjects. Correlation and regression are often confused, perhaps because of the similarity of the mathematics involved, but they have quite different functions.

## Functions

**1. *Correlation.*** This is used to evaluate whether two continuous variables are associated; i.e. do patients with large values of one variable also generally have large values of the other variable, or are perhaps large values of one associated with small values of the other and *vice versa*. Sometimes, there is one variable which correlates with multiple other variables.

**2. *Regression.*** This is used to predict the value of one continuous variable from the other, if the two variables are associated.

## Correlation

Correlation is a statistical method used for quantifying any association between two continuous variables. *Figure 1* shows the correlation between concentrations of sevoflurane, an inhalational anaesthetic agent, and phrenic nerve activity (PNA) in rabbits. It can be seen that PNA was depressed progressively with increasing concentrations of sevoflurane. PNA is a good indicator of the activity of the respiratory control system. Therefore, this figure suggests that sevoflurane causes a dose-dependent depression of respiration.

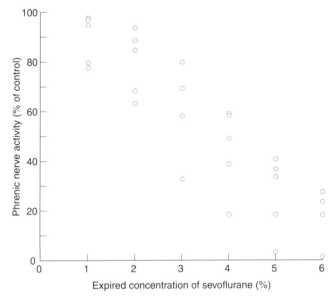

Figure 1. Scattergram showing correlation between phrenic nerve activity (% of control) and concentrations of sevoflurane (%).

**1. _Correlation coefficient._** This is a measure of the degree of 'straight line' association between two continuous variables and is denoted by $r$, which may vary from $-1$ or $+1$.

- If the value of $r$ is _positive_, the two variables are positively correlated – both tend to increase together (_Figure 2(a)_).
- If the value of $r$ is _negative_, the two variables are negatively correlated – one decreases as the other increases (_Figure 2(b)_).
- If $r$ is _zero_ the two variables are uncorrelated (_Figure 2(c)_).

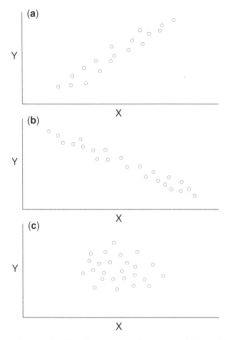

Figure 2. Scattergram showing (a) positive, (b) negative and (c) zero correlation.

**2. _Calculation of r._** There are two types of correlation coefficient, Pearson's $r$ and Spearman's $r_s$.

- _Pearson's $r$_ is used when data are normally distributed.
- _Spearman's rank $r_s$_ is used for non-parametric data.
- They can be calculated by using computer packages which are based on a standard formula. For example, if several values of two variables $x$ and $y$ are known, Pearson's $r$ can be calculated from the formula:

$$r = \sum\{(x-\bar{x})(y-\bar{y})\}/\sqrt{\sum(x-\bar{x})^2 \sum(y-\bar{y})^2}$$

where $x$ and $y$ are the individual values, and $\bar{x}$ and $\bar{y}$ are the mean values of $x$ and $y$ respectively.

**3. _Confidence interval of r._** The 95% confidence interval can be calculated for the correlation in the population, on the assumption that the sample is representative. The calculation requires both variables to be normally distributed.

**4.** *Hypothesis tests for* r. A correlation coefficient can be calculated for any scatter diagram, but hypothesis tests must be used to identify if the association is statistically significant.

- Both variables should be measured in each subject in a random sample of individuals.
- Only one pair of values must be obtained in each individual.
- The null hypothesis is that $r$ is zero.
- At least one variable should have a normal distribution for Pearson's $r$. If not, the data should be transformed, or a test for Spearman's rank $r_s$ should be used.
- The hypothesis test for the significance of $r$ is based on the $t$ distribution.
- The Pearson correlation coefficient table gives the $P$-value for a given $r$ associated with a given sample size.

## Regression

If two variables are associated, regression can predict one from the other only within the range of values in the observed data.

**1.** *Simple linear regression.* Simple linear regression calculates the equation of the 'best' straight line relating one variable to the other.

- The general equation of a regression line is:

$$y = a + bx$$

where $a$ is the value of $y$ when $x = 0$, and $b$ is the slope. This says that each $y$-value is $b$ times the appropriate $x$-value plus or minus a constant increment.
- $y$ is considered as the *response* variable that is always plotted on the vertical, or $y$ axis. $x$ is the *predictor* variable that is always on the horizontal, or $x$ axis.
- The *slope* is an important parameter in regression analysis, as it indicates the degree of the association between two variables. However, the value of $a$ will have no practical meaning in most medical applications, as the $x$ variable can not be anywhere near zero.
- *An example. Figure 3* shows a linear regression between concentrations of sevoflurane and PNA (the same data as *Figure 1*). The regression equation can be expressed as PNA (% of control) $= 106 - 16$ (concentration of sevoflurane). The slope of the fitted line is $-16$, which means that it can be estimated that there is a decrease in PNA of 16% of control for every increase of one unit (%) in concentration of sevoflurane (see *Figure 3*).

**2.** *Assumptions.* The following assumptions should be met before the use of regression analysis:

- the values of $y$ should have a normal distribution for each value of $x$;
- the standard deviation of $y$ about the mean should be approximately the same for each value of $x$;
- the relation between the two variables should be linear;
- both variables may be non-random variables;
- the values of $x$ need not be normally distributed.

When the above assumptions hold, the regression line gives an estimate of the mean values of $y$ for each value of $x$.

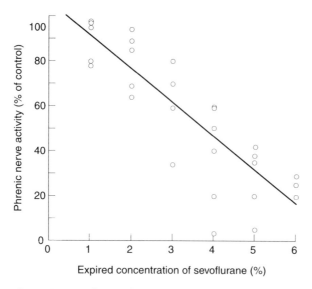

Figure 3. Correlation between concentrations of sevoflurane and phrenic nerve activity. The regression line is $Y = 106 - 16X$ and the correlation coefficient is $r = 0.82$ (data as *Figure 1*).

**3. 95% confidence interval (CI).** The regression line represents an estimate of the average value of $y$ for each value of $x$. The 95% confidence interval (*Figure 4*) encompasses the range of values of $y$ within which one is 95% confident that the true mean of $y$ in the population lies. The CI is narrowest at the mean value of $x$ and becomes wider with increasing distance from the mean. Increasing the sample size narrows, and reducing the sample size, increases the width of the CI.

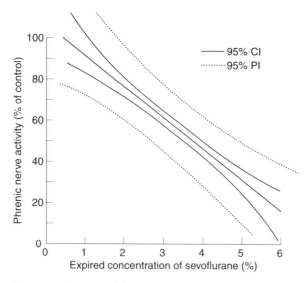

Figure 4. 95% confidence interval for the predicted mean value of y for specified values of x (data as in *Figures 1* and *3*).

**4. 95% prediction interval (PI).** This gives the limits within which one can expect the actual value of y to lie in 95% of future patients. It is much wider than the CI (see *Figure 4*). A very wide prediction interval indicates that for a given value of x there is considerable uncertainty about the value of y and in these circumstances the 95% prediction interval is of little clinical value. The precision of the data, not the sample size, affects the width of 95% prediction interval.

## Multiple linear regression

This technique is used to predict the value of one variable from values of two or more other variables. For example, to predict peak expiratory flow (PEF) from height, weight and age.

**Multiple correlation coefficient ($R^2$).** $R^2$ is the percentage of the variation in the value of y. For example, $R^2 = 22\%$ for the regression between PEF and age means that 22% of the variation in PEF can be accounted for by age.

(a) $R^2$ is exactly the same as $r^2$, the square of the Pearson correlation coefficient, but it should not be interpreted in the same way.

(b) If the regression is significant and the value of $R^2$ is rather small the explanation could be:
- another known or unknown variable is involved;
- the relationship is real, but the data are rather variable;
- the relationship is a false-positive one, resulting in a type I error.

## Steps in the use of correlation and regression analysis

- Draw a scatter diagram to give an indication of any association between two variables;
- Calculate the correlation coefficient ($r$) and if $r$ is statistically significant, simple linear regression analysis can be performed;
- Choose multiple linear regression analysis if one variable is influenced by several variables.

## Further reading

Altman DG. Table B7 – Pearson's correlation coefficient In: Altman DG, (ed). *Practical Statistics for Medical Research*. London: Chapman and Hall. 1991, pp. 528–529.

Armitage P, Berry G. Regression and correlation. In: Armitage P and Berry G, (eds). *Statistical Methods in Medical Research*. 3rd edn. Oxford: Blackwell Scientific Publications, 1994, pp. 141–159.

Godfrey K. Simple linear regression in medical research. In: Bailar JC III, Mosteller F, (eds). *Medical Uses of Statistics*, 2nd edition. Boston: NEJM Book, 1992, pp. 201–231.

## Related topics of interest

Choice of statistical methods, p. 164; Measures of central tendency and dispersion, p. 83; The normal distribution, p. 89; Types of data, p. 74; Logistic regression, p. 152.

# LOGISTIC REGRESSION

*Magnus A. McGee*

In medicine it is common to record the absence or presence of a condition. A variable taking only two values is called a **binary** or dichotomous variable. Logistic regression is used to describe the relationship between a binary variable and known explanatory variables.

## Probability and odds

*1. Absence or presence of a condition.* MacArthur *et al.* reported the prevalence of faecal incontinence in 7,152 mothers, three months after delivery. The method of delivery is grouped into three factors or categories: spontaneous vaginal delivery (natural childbirth); assisted vaginal delivery (where the baby was a breech birth or forceps or vacuum forceps were used) and caesarean section. The total number of participants (n), the number (r) and percentage (%) with faecal incontinence for each method delivery are reported (see *Table 1*).

**Table 1.** The number of mothers by type of delivery and the number and percentage of those with faecal incontinence (FI) three months after giving birth by type of delivery ($n = 7,152$)

| Delivery | Number ($n$) | FI | | Odds $r/(n\text{-}r)$ | Odds ratio odds(delivery)/odds(SVD) |
|---|---|---|---|---|---|
| | | $r$ | (%) | | |
| SVD | 4,964 | 474 | (9.5) | 0.106 | 1 |
| AVD | 1,048 | 132 | (12.6) | 0.144 | 1.37 |
| CS | 1,140 | 84 | (7.4) | 0.080 | 0.75 |
| Total | 7,152 | 690 | (9.6) | 0.107 | |

Abbreviations: SVD, spontaneous vaginal delivery; AVD, assisted vaginal delivery; CS, caesarean section.

*2. Odds.* To describe the data for each method of delivery, the percentage (the probability times one hundred) and the odds are given. The observed percentage with faecal incontinence is approximately 10% and is highest for assisted vaginal delivery. The odds of faecal incontinence being present versus being absent are $690/(7,152 - 690) = 0.11$, approximately one to nine and, again, is highest for assisted vaginal delivery.

*3. Odds ratios.* The best way to compare methods of delivery is to use odds ratios. Here one category, spontaneous vaginal delivery, is defined as the reference category. The other categories are then compared with it. Spontaneous vaginal delivery is selected because it is the most meaningful for purposes of interpretation. (It is also common to select the reference category as the group with the largest number of observations.)

## Statistical knowledge

It is vital to understand what categorical, ordinal, binary and continuous variables are. Any experience already gained using linear regression will help you use logistic regression. Here the dependent variable used in linear regression is replaced by the *log odds*, i.e. the natural logarithm of the odds. To use logistic regression the following pointers will help. Make sure the outcome variable is binary, it should only take one of two values. It will also make analysis easier if it takes the values zero or one.

## Example

Let us look at a logistic regression of the odds of faecal incontinence occurring (the binary outcome variable) given the mode of delivery (the explanatory variable), using the data from *Table 1*. The software package needs to know the name of the outcome variable containing the number having the condition present (r), the total numbers of patients (n), the mode of delivery and that the mode of delivery is a categorical variable.

The results are presented in *Table 2* and mimic the output from the software package. There is one line for all but one category, spontaneous vaginal delivery, the reference category. We already know its odds ratio is one and the odds ratio for the other two categories are relative to it. If the odds ratio is greater than one then the category increases the chances of the complication being present and is considered harmful. If the odds ratio is less than one, it shows the category to be protective. The coefficient is the log odds for the category compared with the reference category and its standard error is also reported. Their ratio is reported in the next column, z-value, with its P-value beside it. Finally the 95% confidence interval for the coefficient, the odds ratio and the 95% confidence interval for the odds ratio are reported.

**Table 2.** Results from a logistic regression of faecal incontinence on method of delivery (n=7152)

| Delivery | Coeff. | Std. Err. | z-ratio | P-value | Coeff. 95% CI | OR | OR 95% CI |
|----------|--------|-----------|---------|---------|---------------|------|-----------|
| AVD | 0.31 | 0.10 | 2.97 | 0.003 | (0.10 , 0.52) | 1.37 | (1.11 , 1.68) |
| CS | −0.28 | 0.12 | −2.30 | 0.022 | (−0.52 , −0.04) | 0.75 | (0.59 , 0.96) |

Abbreviations: Coeff, coefficient; CI, confidence interval; OR, odds ratio; AVD, assisted vaginal delivery; CS, caesarean section.

The coefficients for the two methods of delivery suggest that assisted vaginal delivery (odds ratio = 1.37) may increase the chance of faecal incontinence while caesarean section (odds ratio = 0.75) decreases it. The odds ratios here are the same as those in *Table 1*. This is true when there is only one explanatory variable in the logistic regression. Whether assisted vaginal delivery or caesarean section changes the odds of faecal incontinence relative to spontaneous vaginal delivery is shown by the fact that the odds ratio confidence intervals do not contain one. Similarly the coefficient confidence intervals do not contain zero. Further confirmation is given by the two P-values for delivery, which test assisted vaginal delivery and caesarean section versus spontaneous vaginal delivery respectively. The overall effect of delivery is left to 'Further reading'. The confidence interval for the odds of faecal incontinence with assisted vaginal delivery relative to spontaneous vaginal delivery confirms that there is at least an 11% greater chance (95% CI from 1.11 to 1.68) of reporting faecal incontinence after assisted vaginal delivery.

## Acknowledgements

The Health Services Research Unit receives core funding from the Chief Scientists Office of the Scottish Executive Health Department. The views expressed in this topic are those of the author and not necessarily those of the Department.

## Further reading

Clayton D, Hills M. *Statistical Models in Epidemiology.* Oxford: Oxford University Press, 1993.

Hosmer DW, Lemeshow S. *Applied Logistic Regression.* New York: John Wiley & Sons, 1989.

MacArthur C, Glazner CMA, Wilson PD, Herbison GP, Gee H, Lang GD, Lancashire R. Obstetric practice and faecal incontinence three months after delivery. *British Journal of Obstetrics and Gynaecology* 2001; **108:** 678–683.

# SURVIVAL DATA

*Graeme MacLennan*

## General concepts

**1. Survival analysis.** This is a set of statistical techniques used when the primary outcome of interest is the time between patients' entry into a study and a subsequent outcome. In medical applications this outcome is usually death, but not always. For example, the outcome may be time to recurrence.

**2. Survival time.**

(a) *Calculation.* Survival time is calculated as the time elapsing between some natural starting point (baseline) and the outcome of interest.

(b) *Types of data.* To understand the difficulties of using survival time in a study, let us consider a hypothetical cohort of six patients receiving a new surgical procedure for treatment of colorectal cancer. The study started on 1 January. Recruitment lasted for 1 month and the patients were followed up until the end of the year *(Figure 1)*.

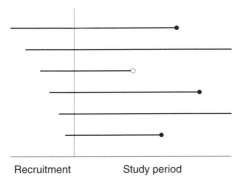

Recruitment          Study period

Figure 1. Survival data.

- In *Figure 1* we can see that three of the patients died before the end of follow-up (black circles).
- However, two of the patients survived until at least the end of the study period.
- One patient (white circle) was somehow lost to follow up; for example, the patient may have died from some non-colorectal-cancer-related cause or may have moved from the area.
- Patients who have survived and patients who are lost to follow up are patients who have not experienced the outcome of interest during the period of observation. Such data are said to be right censored. Although data can be left censored, most survival data are right censored, and from here on, all censored data referred to will be right censored.

- At the last point of follow-up such patients were known not to have experienced the outcome of interest, so we have some information on survival time, but not exact survival time. Because of this, standard methods (e.g. logistic regression on the dead/alive outcome, or a comparison of mean survival times), are not valid. So, we need to use statistical techniques developed specifically to present and analyse such data.

**3. Cumulative probabilities of patients' survival.** In medical studies we are frequently interested in survival after some clinical intervention. There are two statistical techniques that give cumulative probabilities of patients' survival after intervention.

*(a) Life tables*
- In the life table approach, survival times are grouped into convenient intervals. This is useful if only approximate survival times are available.
- Also, it may be more appropriate to use life table methods with large samples.

*(b) Kaplan–Meier survival curve*
- Kaplan–Meier can be used with any sample size, but is useful when small sample sizes mean that satisfactory grouping is unfeasible, or when exact survival times are known.

Both techniques use simple methods for calculating the survival probabilities that are easily implemented through statistics packages. The techniques will be illustrated using the following example.

# Worked example 1

Data on 50 patients undergoing renal replacement therapy over 78 months were collected. Each patient was categorized as low ($n=24$) or high risk ($n=26$). The primary outcome was the survival time after commencing renal replacement therapy until death. In addition to the survival time in days, data were collected on the sex of the patient and on whether the patient had a transplant during the study period.

# Life tables

**1. A life table.** *Table 1* contains information on survival for the whole cohort of 50 patients. In this example, the survival times have been grouped into 6-month periods for convenience. In some instances though, data are only collected at fixed time intervals; such situations do arise. *Table 1* is adapted from SPSS computer software output.

**2. Calculation.** From *Table 1*, we can see that the number of observed cases in the first time period was 50. So, we say that $O_1 = 50$. However, there were two censored patients in this time period, $C_1 = 2$. The probability of death in the time period needs to account for this.

(a) *The number exposed to the risk of death* ($E_x$)
- The number exposed to the risk of death in any time period $x$ is defined as

$$E_x = O_x - \frac{C_x}{2}$$

**Table 1.** Life table estimates of survival for renal replacement therapy cohort

| Interval start time | Time period $x$ | Number entering this interval $O_x$ | Number withdrawn during interval $C_x$ | Number exposed to risk $E_x$ | Number of terminal events $d_x$ | Proportion dead $q_x$ | Proportion surviving $p_x$ | Cumulative proportion surviving at end $S_x$ |
|---|---|---|---|---|---|---|---|---|
| 0 | 1 | 50 | 2 | 49.0 | 9 | 0.1837 | 0.8163 | 0.8163 |
| 6 | 2 | 39 | 1 | 38.5 | 2 | 0.0519 | 0.9481 | 0.7739 |
| 12 | 3 | 36 | 1 | 35.5 | 4 | 0.1127 | 0.8873 | 0.6867 |
| 18 | 4 | 31 | 1 | 30.5 | 2 | 0.0656 | 0.9344 | 0.6417 |
| 24 | 5 | 28 | 2 | 27.0 | 2 | 0.0741 | 0.9259 | 0.5942 |
| 30 | 6 | 24 | 3 | 22.5 | 1 | 0.0444 | 0.9556 | 0.5677 |
| 36 | 7 | 20 | 6 | 17.0 | 2 | 0.1176 | 0.8824 | 0.501 |
| 42 | 8 | 12 | 4 | 10.0 | 0 | 0.0 | 1.0 | 0.501 |
| 48+ | 9 | 8 | 6 | 5.0 | 2 | 0.4 | 0.6 | 0.3006 |

So, from *Table 1*, we can see that the $E_1$ is given by

$$E_1 = O_1 - \frac{C_1}{2} = 50 - \frac{2}{2} = 49$$

- Why divide the number of censored cases by a half? Well, one of the assumptions of the life table method is that the patients withdraw *uniformly* throughout the time period. So, on average, patients that are censored are under observation for only half of the time period and the calculations for probability of death (and survival) need to reflect this. See Further reading for further details.

(b) *Probability of death* $(q_x)$. The number of deaths divided by the number of patients at risk in a time period $x$ gives the probability of death in that time period, $q_x = d_x / E_x$, for the first time period

$$q_1 = d_1 / E_1 = 9/49 = 0.1837$$

There was an 18% chance of death in the first 6 months.

(c) *Probability of survival* $(p_x)$. The probability of survival, $p_x$ is given by $1 - q_x$. For the first 6 months the survival probability was

$$p_1 = 1 - 0.1837 = 0.8163 \text{ or } 82\%$$

(d) *Cumulative probability of survival* $(S_x)$. The final column in the table contains the estimated cumulative probability of survival to the end of each time period. For a patient to have survived a year, the patient must have survived the first 6 months and the second 6 months. The estimated probability of this occurring is

$$(p_1)(p_2) = 0.8163 \times 0.9481 = 0.7739$$

So patients had a 77% chance of surviving until the end of the second period. This is extended for each time period. The estimated probability for having survived 18 months is given by:

$$(p_1)(p_2)(p_3) = 0.8163 \times 0.9481 \times 0.8873 = 0.6867$$

This is repeated until the end of the last time period. From the table above the estimated probability of 4-year survival was 50% (survival of time period 8).

**3. Statistical software.** Software packages do these laborious calculations at the click of a button. Each package will produce additional life table statistics (and standard errors) that can be read about in the relevant manuals.

## Kaplan–Meier survival curves

**1. Advantages.** The life table approach suffers from the same limitation as relative frequency tables, which is a loss of precision due to the grouping of data. The Kaplan–Meier Product Limit method can be thought of as a special case of the life table method where time intervals are arbitrarily small, and a time interval will only contain patients that have exactly the same survival time.

**2. The Kaplan–Meier procedure.**

(a) *Survival time between the two groups.* In the following example the renal replacement patients were split into two groups, one high and one low risk. The

Kaplan–Meier procedure from SPSS was used to investigate differences in survival time (in days) between the two groups of patients. *Tables 2 and 3 are* adapted from SPSS output.

**Table 2.** KM estimates for high-risk renal replacement therapy patients

| Time | Status | Number at risk $n_t$ | Number of deaths $d_t$ | Probability of survival $p_t = 1 - d_t/n_t$ | Cumulative survival $S_t$ |
|------|--------|------|------|------|------|
| 1 | DEAD | 26 | 1 | 0.9615 | 0.9615 |
| 7 | DEAD | 25 | 1 | 0.9600 | 0.9231 |
| 17 | DEAD | 24 | 1 | 0.9583 | 0.8846 |
| 32 | DEAD | 23 | 1 | 0.9565 | 0.8462 |
| 49 | DEAD | 22 | 1 | 0.9545 | 0.8077 |
| 96 | DEAD | 21 | 1 | 0.9524 | 0.7692 |
| 122 | DEAD | 20 | 1 | 0.9500 | 0.7308 |
| 125 | DEAD | 19 | 1 | 0.9474 | 0.6923 |
| 168 | DEAD | 18 | 1 | 0.9444 | 0.6538 |
| 241 | DEAD | 17 | 1 | 0.9412 | 0.6154 |
| 271 | DEAD | 16 | 1 | 0.9375 | 0.5769 |
| 375 | DEAD | 15 | 1 | 0.9333 | 0.5385 |
| 378 | DEAD | 14 | 1 | 0.9286 | 0.5 |
| 389 | ALIVE | 13 | 0 | | |
| 451 | DEAD | 12 | 1 | 0.9167 | 0.4583 |
| 488 | DEAD | 11 | 1 | 0.9091 | 0.4167 |
| 558 | DEAD | 10 | 1 | 0.9000 | 0.375 |
| 599 | DEAD | 9 | 1 | 0.8889 | 0.3333 |
| 684 | ALIVE | 8 | 0 | | |
| 1158 | DEAD | 7 | 1 | 0.8571 | 0.2857 |
| 1218 | ALIVE | 6 | 0 | | |
| 1308 | ALIVE | 5 | 0 | | |
| 1713 | DEAD | 4 | 1 | 0.7500 | 0.2143 |
| 2180 | ALIVE | 3 | 0 | | |
| 2240 | DEAD | 2 | 1 | 0.5000 | 0.1071 |
| 2638 | ALIVE | 1 | 0 | | |

(b) *The Kaplan–Meier estimates*
- The column of interest is the last column in these tables, which gives the cumulative survival estimates, also known as the Kaplan–Meier or product limit estimates.
- The method for calculating Kaplan–Meier estimates is very similar to that of the life table estimates, but the reasoning behind the method is beyond the scope of this text.

(c) *A Kaplan–Meier survival curve*
- The Kaplan–Meier estimates of survival can also be represented graphically.
- A Kaplan–Meier survival curve has time on the *x-axis* and the Kaplan–Meier estimates on the *y-axis*. The survival curves in *Figure 2* show the cumulative survival probabilities of the renal replacement therapy patients from the high- and low-risk groups.

**Table 3.** KM estimates for low-risk renal replacement therapy patients

| Time | Status | Number at risk $n_t$ | Number of deaths $d_t$ | Probability of survival $p_t = 1 - d_t/n_t$ | Cumulative survival $S_t$ |
|---|---|---|---|---|---|
| 48 | ALIVE | 24 | 0 | | |
| 147 | ALIVE | 23 | 0 | | |
| 737 | ALIVE | 22 | 0 | | |
| 758 | DEAD | 21 | 1 | 0.9524 | 0.9524 |
| 789 | ALIVE | 20 | 0 | | |
| 810 | DEAD | 19 | 1 | 0.9474 | 0.9023 |
| 945 | ALIVE | 18 | 0 | | |
| 948 | DEAD | 17 | 1 | 0.9412 | 0.8492 |
| 972 | ALIVE | 16 | 0 | | |
| 1021 | ALIVE | 15 | 0 | | |
| 1096 | ALIVE | 14 | 0 | | |
| 1099 | ALIVE | 13 | 0 | | |
| 1119 | DEAD | 12 | 1 | 0.9167 | 0.7784 |
| 1188 | ALIVE | 11 | 0 | | |
| 1190 | ALIVE | 10 | 0 | | |
| 1194 | ALIVE | 9 | 0 | | |
| 1246 | ALIVE | 8 | 0 | | |
| 1335 | ALIVE | 7 | 0 | | |
| 1429 | ALIVE | 6 | 0 | | |
| 1471 | ALIVE | 5 | 0 | | |
| 1747 | ALIVE | 4 | 0 | | |
| 2090 | ALIVE | 3 | 0 | | |
| 2105 | ALIVE | 2 | 0 | | |
| 2255 | ALIVE | 1 | 0 | | |

- The *steps* in the curve indicate deaths and the *ticks* on the curve indicate the censored times of survivors.
- A summary statistic that can be read from the graph (and is provided by the computer package) is the *median survival time*. (*Note*: If there were no censored data (everyone died), the median would just be the middle observation of the ranked survival times.) This can be read by extending a horizontal line from the vertical axis at $P = 0.5$ until the curve is met, and then extending this line to the horizontal axis. This gives the median survival time (see the dashed line on graph) (see *Figure 2*). For the high-risk group, the median survival time was 378 days. Because more than 50% of the low-risk group were censored (i.e. still alive), the median survival time was not calculated.
- At the end of the study period 77% (20/26) of patients in the high-risk group had died compared to 17% (4/24) in the low-risk group. It therefore appears that there was a difference in survival between the two groups. How can we test this difference statistically? Because of the censored observations, the Chi squared test (see Chi squared test, p. 140) is not valid. In such situations, the log rank test can be used.

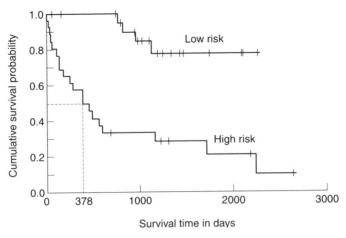

Figure 2. Kaplan–Meier survival curves for low- and high-risk renal replacement therapy patients.

## Log rank test

The log rank test is a non-parametric test that can be used to compare the difference in survival curves between two or more groups (*Table 4*).

**Table 4.** Results of log rank test

|          | Statistic | Df | P-value  |
| -------- | --------- | -- | -------- |
| Log rank | 17.71     | 1  | <0.001   |

*Question:* Was the survival curve in the high-risk group significantly different from that of the low-risk group?

*Null hypothesis:* No difference between the survival curves.

*Alternative hypothesis:* There is a difference between survival curves.

- The log rank statistic follows a chi-square distribution with 1 degree of freedom under the null hypothesis of no difference between the survival curves. Here we can see that the test statistic is significant ($P<0.001$). This highlights that the difference between the survival rates is unlikely to be due to chance and we therefore reject the null hypothesis and conclude that the high-risk group have less chance of survival.
- The test can be extended to compare $k>2$ groups, with the test statistic having $k-1$ degrees of freedom.

## Hazard ratio

**1. *Background.*** The log rank test does not allow us to test for the independent effects of a number of factors on survival time. A regression technique that facilitates such modelling is Cox Proportional Hazards modelling.

**2. Definition.**

(a) *Hazard.* The hazard is the risk that a patient has at a certain time point of experiencing the outcome of interest (usually risk of death), given that they have not experienced it already.

(b) *Hazard ratio.* The hazard ratio is interpreted in a similar way as the odds ratio from logistic regression (see topic 'Logistic regression' p. 152). A hazard ratio greater than one indicates an increased risk, whilst less than one indicates a decreased risk. If the confidence interval for the hazard ratio straddles one, then it can be said to be statistically non-significant.

**3. Calculation model.** Cox Proportional Hazards models the underlying hazard rate as a function of a set of independent variables (factors) rather than the actual survival times.

**4. An example.** To highlight this in practice, we shall look again at the 50 renal replacement patients. We wish to investigate the effects of sex, risk group and whether the patient received a kidney transplant on the probability of survival (*Table 5*).

**Table 5.** Results from Cox Proportional Hazards Model

| Variable | Estimated coefficient | Standard error | *P*-value | Hazard ratio | 95% confidence interval |
|---|---|---|---|---|---|
| Risk (0 = low, 1 = high) | 1.43 | 0.15 | 0.006 | 4.18 | (1.37–13.09) |
| Transplant (0 = no, 1 = yes) | −1.74 | 0.63 | 0.014 | 0.18 | (0.05–0.60) |
| Sex (0 = male, 1 = female) | 0.53 | 0.47 | 0.258 | 1.16 | (0.68–4.29) |

**5. Interpretation.**

(a) *Baseline.* In the model used, the baseline hazard was for male, low-risk, non-transplant patients. So, from the table above we can immediately see that the patients in the high-risk groups were much less likely to survive than those in the low-risk group when accounting for sex and transplant status.

(b) *Hazard ratio.* In fact, the patients in the high-risk group were four times (hazard ratio = 4.18) more likely to die than the low-risk group. Also, we can see that patients who had a transplant were more likely to survive (hazard ratio = 0.18). The confidence interval for the hazard ratio for sex includes one and is non-significant, so there was no difference in survival between males and females.

**Acknowledgement**
The Health Services Research Unit receives core funding from the Chief Scientists Office of the Scottish Executive Health Department. The views expressed in this topic are those of the author and not necessarily those of the Department.

# Further reading

Altman DG. *Practical Statistics for Medical Research*. London: Chapman & Hall, 1991.

Bland JM, Altman DG. Time to event (survival) data. *British Medical Journal* 1997; **317**: 468–469.

Bland M. *An Introduction to Medical Statistics,* 2nd edn. Oxford: Oxford Medical Publications, 1995.

Cox DR, Oakes D. *Analysis of Survival Data*. London: Chapman & Hall, 1984.

# Related topics of interest

Chi squared and Fisher's exact test, p. 140; Logistic regression, p. 152.

# CHOICE OF STATISTICAL METHODS

*Fang Gao Smith, John E. Smith*

The research question one asks determines the design of the study, the number of groups, the type of data, etc. These factors, in turn, define the statistical method that is needed. This topic is a cookbook summarizing the appropriate statistical tests to use when answering the most commonly asked research questions.

## Research questions

*1. **Comparison.*** 'Is there a difference between two or more sets of observations in the same group, or in two groups, or in more than two groups?' These questions may be answered using comparison statistical analysis (see *Table 1*).

*2. **Association and prediction.*** 'Is there an association between variables or can this variable predict another variable?' These questions may be answered using association statistical analysis (see *Table 2*).

## Which comparison test? (*Table 1*)

*1. **Types of data.*** The data may be numerical (quantitative) or categorical (qualitative).

| | NUMERICAL | | CATEGORICAL | |
|---|---|---|---|---|
| | Normal distribution | Non-normal distribution | Ordinal | Nominal |
| **COMPARING PAIRED GROUPS** | | | | |
| **2 groups** | Paired *t*-test | Wilcoxon matched pairs signed rank sum test | | McNemar test |
| **>2 groups** | Repeated measures ANOVA | Friedman's test | | Cochran Q test |
| **COMPARING INDEPENDENT GROUPS** | | | | |
| **2 groups** | Unpaired *t*-test | Mann-Whitney U test | | Chi squared test Fisher's exact test |
| **>2 groups** | One-way ANOVA | Kruskal-Wallis (rank) ANOVA | | Chi squared test |

Table 1. Choice of statistical methods for comparisons between groups.

**2. *Distribution of numerical data.*** Normally distributed data can be analysed using parametric tests. Non-normal numerical data can be analysed in the same way as ordinal categorical data using non-parametric tests.

**3. *Paired or independent data.*** Two or more paired groups occur when two or more sets of observations are made on the same, single sample of individuals. Two groups may be compared using, for example, the paired *t*-test or the Wilcoxon matched pairs signed rank sum test whereas more than two groups would require repeated measures ANOVA or Friedman's test. Independent comparisons involve unrelated groups of patients. For example, two independent groups might be compared using unpaired *t*-test whereas more than two groups might be compared using one-way ANOVA

## Which association test? (*Table 2*)

| | | VARIABLE 1 | | | |
|---|---|---|---|---|---|
| | | NUMERICAL | | CATEGORICAL | |
| | | Normal | Non-normal | Ordinal | Nominal |
| VARIABLE 2 — NUMERICAL | Normal | regression correlation | regression rank correlation | rank correlation | analysis of variance |
| VARIABLE 2 — NUMERICAL | Non-normal | regression rank correlation | rank correlation | rank correlation | Kruskal-Wallis test |
| VARIABLE 2 — CATEGORICAL | Ordinal | rank correlation | rank correlation | rank correlation | Kruskal-Wallis test |
| VARIABLE 2 — CATEGORICAL | Nominal | analysis of variance | Kruskal-Wallis test | Kruskal-Wallis test | chi squared test |

Table 2. Choice of statistical methods for associations between two variables (variable 1 and variable 2).

**1. *Types of data.*** Again, the data may be numerical or categorical.

**2. *Distribution of numerical data.*** When both numerical variables are normally distributed, the data can be analysed for correlation using Pearson's *r*, whereas if one or both variables are non-normally distributed, Spearman's *r* is appropriate.

**3. *Categorical data.*** The appropriate tests for categorical data can be seen in *Table 2*. For example, if both variables are ordinal then Spearman's rank correlation can be used whereas if both variables are nominal, chi squared test is necessary.

## Algorithms

- The algorithms (see *Table 1–2*) should only be used as general guides for the selection of the most appropriate test.
- In practice, there may be more than one statistical approach to the results of even a simple clinical trial. Hence, different statisticians might recommend different tests for the analysis of the same data ( just as different clinicians may

recommend different treatments for a particular disease). For example, one statistician may have very strict criteria for the acceptance of the assumption of normality while another statistician may seldom use non-parametric tests.

- Readers should refer to the appropriate topics in this book to understand the assumptions for the various tests and common difficulties.

## Further reading

Altman DG. Comparing groups – continuous data and categorical data. In: Altman DG, (ed). *Practical Statistics For Medical Research*. London: Chapman and Hall, 1991; 179–276.

Bland M. Choosing the statistical method. In: Bland M. *An Introduction to Medical Statistics*. Oxford: Oxford Medical Publication, 1995; 254–264.

## Related topics of interest

Analysis of variance (ANOVA), p. 133; Chi square and Fisher's exact test, p. 140; Correlation and regression, p. 147; Descriptive statistics and inferential statistics, p. 72; Mann–Whitney U test, p. 128; Student's *t* test, p. 110; Types of data, p. 74; Wilcoxon matched pairs signed rank sum test, p. 124.

# SYSTEMATIC REVIEWS AND META-ANALYSIS
*Martin Wildman*

## The need for summaries of the research literature

- The delivery of health care requires clinicians to choose the best treatments for their patients. This requires expertise in the use of information, identifying key conclusions from a morass of available evidence.
- Researchers also need to have a thorough and critical understanding of previous research in the field in which a new study is planned.
- Systematic reviews and meta-analysis are intended to integrate the mass of research evidence relevant to a particular question. An understanding of the strengths and weaknesses of systematic reviews and meta-analysis is crucial for a clinician involved in research or in service delivery.

## Definitions

Systematic reviews and meta-analysis both require an exhaustive, explicit and reproducible identification of all evidence relating to the subject of the review.

*1. Meta-analysis.* A meta-analysis is a particular type of systematic review in which the measures of effect from individual studies are combined into a single overall measure that synthesizes the findings from the studies identified. Meta-analysis is particularly well suited to combining data from randomized controlled trials (RCTs) and the Cochrane Collaboration have specialized in this.

*2. Systematic review.* In a systematic review the results from the individual studies are typically not combined into a single summary measure of effect, but may be presented in tables or narrative format.

## Features

*1. The science of evidence synthesis.* In the past an 'expert' might write a (non-systematic) review by drawing conclusions from the results of studies with which the author was familiar. The conclusions would typically be heavily biased by the studies that happened to be selected, and another expert might write a review addressing the same question but drawing on different studies and reaching a different conclusion. A systematic review is intended to avoid such bias by rigorously identifying all studies relevant to a specific question.

*2. Secondary research.* A transparent and reproducible method is then used to draw conclusions about how the results of individual studies lead to the message to be taken from the research base as a whole. This discipline of primary study assimilation is known as secondary research. Secondary research mirrors primary research in that both of them frame a focused question and develop a reproducible method designed to answer that question.

*3. Ideal form.* In their ideal form, systematic reviews and meta-analysis rigorously identify, appraise, and synthesize evidence using well-defined methods that would allow a second reviewer approaching the same question to identify the same studies and reach a similar conclusion. In practice, this is not always the case.

# Methods

A systematic review and a meta-analysis involve the following important stages:

- Formulating an explicit review question.
- Formulating an explicit search strategy.
- Developing an explicit set of criteria for including and excluding studies.
- Synthesizing results.

**1. *Formulating an explicit review question.*** This is a crucial stage in planning a systematic review, just as the formulation of a hypothesis is crucial to the design of primary research. Typically a question will have *three parts*:

(a) Definition of the *population* involved.
(b) Definition of the *intervention* about which evidence is sought.
(c) Definition of the *outcome* of interest.

Consider, for example, a question about the effectiveness of non-invasive ventilation in patients with acute respiratory failure due to chronic obstructive pulmonary disease (COPD).

(a) *The population* would be patients admitted to hospital with acute respiratory failure due to COPD.
(b) *The intervention* would be non-invasive ventilation.
(c) *The outcome* might be hospital mortality.

Formulating an explicit question will require a detailed understanding of the area under consideration, so that definitions anticipate the variety that will be encountered in the literature and it is clear in advance which studies should be included or excluded.

**2. *Formulating an explicit search strategy.*** The question that the systematic review addresses will determine the type of studies that are sought. For example, a question about *effectiveness* will typically involve a search for randomized controlled trials. A question about *prognosis* would be likely to require a search for observational cohort studies.

(a) *Literature search.* The identification of relevant publications seeks to be exhaustive. The aim is to reduce bias in the studies selected. Medline is the largest biomedical research literature database; however, there are many other databases with differences in emphasis and scope. The systematic identification of all available studies requires considerable expertise and information scientists (such as librarians) would typically give advice and support in the development of search strategies and the identification of the databases to use.
(b) *Publication bias in randomized controlled trials.* In studies of effectiveness publication bias is important. Publication bias is the tendency for studies concerning the effectiveness of an intervention or drug to be more likely to be published if they give a positive result. For example, a study carried out in a non-English-speaking country might be more likely to be published in a mainstream English language journal if it gives a positive result, but may be published in a foreign language journal if it is negative. A search strategy that only identified English articles would be biased towards finding studies showing a positive result.

(c) *Publication bias in cohort studies.* It should be remembered that, though publication bias has been investigated and confirmed as a problem in RCTs, there is less evidence about publication bias in other study designs. For example, in cohort studies designed to determine prognosis, the pressures against publication may be more to do with size and quality. Thus in the prognostic literature it may be small methodologically flawed studies that are unpublished or published in obscure foreign language journals. Such studies may well be of inadequate quality to inform the question that is the basis of the review. Thus, in questions answered by cohort studies, a search failing to identify all studies may be less likely to produce an important bias in the results of the review.

**3. *Developing an explicit set of criteria for including and excluding studies.*** It is important that explicit criteria are developed *a priori* to decide which studies should be included or excluded. The process of deciding which studies to include should include critical appraisal of the internal validity of studies using an approach that pays attention to the key aspects of design that are pertinent to the study in question. For example, in randomized controlled trials looking at questions of effectiveness, key aspects of quality concern randomization and blinding. Inadequate blinding has been shown to be associated with distorted measures of effect. Critical appraisal tools for the different types of study have been published (see Further reading).

**4. *Synthesizing results.*** Meta-analysis is particularly relevant in studies of effectiveness where an active treatment is compared to placebo in a randomized controlled trial. The patients in one trial are not directly compared with another but each trial is analysed separately with summary statistics calculated for each trial. The summary statistics are then added together in the meta-analysis to give a summary measure of effect. Systematic identification of other types of evidence may not lend itself to combination in this way. In these cases the results might be summarized in tables that describe and comment upon the findings of the systematically identified studies.

## Using systematic reviews and meta-analysis

**1. *Assessing the quality.*** Just as assessing quality is important for researchers using individual studies to produce systematic reviews, so quality assessment is important in assessing systematic reviews or meta-analysis used to inform decision-making. Guidelines highlighting the relevant quality criteria have been published (see Further reading).

**2. *Using clinical expertise to interpret the results.*** The conclusions of systematic reviews and the summary measure of effect in meta-analysis should always be interpreted using the clinical expertise of the practitioner. Meta-analysis aiming to answer the same question and drawing on similar studies can produce conflicting results (see Further reading) and a meta-analysis of small trials may be contradicted by subsequent large randomized controlled trials (see Further reading).

**3. *Compendia of the relevant trials.*** Given the potential for systematic reviews and meta-analysis to produce inconsistent results, practitioners might perhaps best consider these reviews as compendia of the relevant trials. They can then look critically both at the individual studies and the overall findings of the review before drawing their own conclusions about the overall message to be drawn from a body of evidence.

## Further reading

Hopayian K. The need for caution in interpreting high quality systematic reviews. *British Medical Journal* 2001; **323:** 681–684.

LeLorier J, Gregoire G, Benhaddad A, Lapierre J, Derderian F. Discrepancies between meta-analyses and subsequent large randomised, controlled trials. *The New England Journal of Medicine* 1997; **337:** 536–542.

Moher D, Cook DJ, Eastwood S, Olkin I, Rennie D, Stroup DF. Improving the quality of reports of meta-analyses of randomised controlled trials: the QUOROM statement. *Lancet* 1999; **354:** 1896–1900.

Sacket DL, Straus SE, Richardson WS, Rosenberg W, Haynes RB. *Evidence-Based Medicine. How to practice and Teach EBM.* 2nd edn, Edinburgh: Churchill Livingstone, 2000.

## Related topics of interest

Conducting clinical trials, p. 44; Randomization, p. 40; Literature searching, p. 11.

# SENSITIVITY AND SPECIFICITY

*Somnath Chatterjee*

Clinical and laboratory tests are often used in medicine to help establish a diagnosis. Clinicians need to know how accurate their tests are in diagnosing the true disease status of the patient. For example, how often does an abnormal cervical smear (positive test) indicate that the patient has neoplasia of the cervix (positive disease) and how often does a normal cervical smear (negative test) indicate that the patient does not have neoplasia of the cervix (negative disease)? *Table 1* illustrates the relationship between these possibilities.

**Table 1.** The relationship between cervical smear results and the true disease status in 227 patients with possible neoplasia of the cervix

| Smear test | Neoplasia of the cervix | | Total |
| | Present (+) | Absent (−) | |
|---|---|---|---|
| Abnormal (+) | 87 | 65 | 152 |
| Normal (−) | 12 | 63 | 75 |
| **Total** | **99** | **128** | **227** |

## True and false positives and negatives

Some patients who had a positive cervical smear did have neoplasia (true positives), but some were found, after further investigations, not to have neoplasia (false positives; *Table 2*). Some patients who had a normal cervical smear did not have the disease (true negatives), but some were found, at a later date, to have neoplasia of the cervix (false negatives).

**Table 2.** True and false positives and negatives

| Diagnostic test | True disease status | |
| | +ve | −ve |
|---|---|---|
| +ve | True positive | False positive |
| −ve | False negative | True negative |

## Sensitivity

The sensitivity of a test is the proportion of disease positives that are correctly identified by the test.

The sensitivity of a test is its true-positive rate, and is expressed as the ratio of true-positive results to all of those with the disease [true positive/(true positive + false negative)]. The sensitivity of the cervical smear test in diagnosing carcinoma of the cervix using the data of *Table 1*, is 87/87 + 12 = 88%. Hence, 88% of patients with abnormal cervical smears will have carcinoma of the cervix.

## Specificity

The specificity of a test is the proportion of disease negatives that are correctly identified by the test.

The specificity of a test is its true-negative rate, and is expressed as the ratio of true-negative results to all those without disease [true negative/(true negative + false positive)]. The specificity of the cervical smear in diagnosing carcinoma of the cervix is 49% (63/63 + 65). Hence, 49% of patients with a normal cervical smear will not have carcinoma.

It may be concluded that when the cervical smear is used as a diagnostic test for neoplasia of the cervix, it has a high sensitivity, because it identifies many true positives. However, it has a relatively low specificity because it does not exclude enough women who do not have neoplasia (it produces many false positives).

## Clinical uses of sensitivity and specificity

Tests with high sensitivity are often used as screening tests as they help to identify true diseases. Tests with high specificity are used as confirmatory tests and are sometimes applied to a group identified by a screening test in order to decrease the number of false-positive results.

## Positive predictive value (PPV)

When a clinician uses a diagnostic test, he or she needs to know how likely the test is to give the correct diagnosis.

The probability that a subject who is test positive will be a true disease positive (the positive predictive value) is the ratio of a true disease positive tests to all positive tests [true positive/(true positive + false positive)]. The positive predictive value of the cervical smear test for carcinoma of the cervix is 87/87 + 65 = 57%.

## Negative predictive value (NPV)

The probability that a subject who is test negative will be a true disease negative (the negative predictive value) is the ratio of the true disease negative to all negative tests [true negative/(true negative + false negative)]. The negative predictive value of the cervical smear test for carcinoma of the cervix is 63/63 + 12 = 84%.

Positive and negative predictive values give a direct assessment of the usefulness of a test in clinical practice.

## Further reading

Altman DG. Diagnostic tests. In: Altman DG (ed). *Practical Statistics for Medical Research.* London: Chapman & Hall, 1991, pp. 409–418.

Sykes MK, Vickers MD, Hull CJ. Radionuclides and their use in clinical measurement. In: Sykes MK, Vickers MD, Hull CJ (eds). *Principles of Measurement and Monitoring in Anaesthesia and Intensive Care,* 3rd edn. London: Blackwell Scientific Publications, 1991, pp. 118–139.

## Related topics of interest

Data collection, p. 64; Laboratory research, p. 17; Measurements, p. 68.

# GIVING A PRESENTATION

*Richard Steyn*

Scientific communication is extremely important if we are to share the results, conclusions and information we have derived from our work. The two main forms of scientific communication are written publications and oral presentations. An oral presentation can be a daunting challenge. The skills required are seldom inherited and sometimes the standard of presentation is poor. However, presentation skills can be learned and then consolidated by practice and rehearsal. Good presentation will not only improve the dissemination of your results but will also enhance your reputation.

## Preparation

1. ***General preparation.*** General personal preparation is important long before considering any individual presentation. When you attend any presentation or lecture consider why you enjoyed or disliked it. Did it interest you or bore you? How was your attention captured and held?

(a) *Consider the audience.* All presentations should be selected and tailored to the audience. Find out ahead of time:
   - what is the purpose of the meeting;
   - who the audience is;
   - how many people will be present;
   - what are their backgrounds;
   - what interest do they have in your presentation.

(b) *Plan your presentation.* Confidence in presentation results from knowing your subject, having your presentation ready and having the right materials to support it. All presentations should be tailored to the time available. However important the information, if too much is presented in too short a time the information will be lost. Decide first what you will leave out, not what you will include. Oral presentations are best used to give an overview of the subject, creating interest. Avoid padding out a presentation with extra information as your audience will actually remember less. The presentation should cover the following.
   - Why was the project undertaken – what were the hypothesis and objective? Give a clear rationale for the study and stress its relevance to current literature/knowledge.
   - What was done – give a clear outline (not details) of the methods. Are the methods supported by current thinking? Ensure that appropriate statistics are used.
   - What was learned – summarize the results emphasizing the main points and relate them to the objective. If the results include large amounts of data then it is useful to select a limited amount and present it in a simple format; more detail can be provided in a handout or as a reference or when answering questions.
   - What does it mean – conclusions should reiterate the main points and any application or relevance for future practice should be clearly stated.

(c) *Visual aids.* The visual aids selected for your presentation should be appropriate for the audience. Computer presentations and graphics are now almost mandatory. Overhead acetates and flip-charts are not usually appropriate for a large audience. Always keep in mind the following questions:

- **Number** of slides – too many or too few? A useful rule of thumb is one slide a minute.
- **Quality** appropriate? The colours and background well-chosen? The font size readable? Concise, neat, well-spaced?
- **Content** appropriate? Do they support or distract the presentation? Is each slide relevant for that part of the talk? Is there a balance between text, photographs, illustrations and tables? Do they 'signpost' and act as an outline for your talk?
- Never apologise for a slide – if the slide is not right it should be re-prepared.

**2. Personal preparation.**

(d) *Rehearsal.*
- Rehearse and practice your presentation in private many times to improve your performance.
- Rehearse and practice in front of colleagues to give you confidence.
- Ensure that you are familiar with your slide set and visual aids.
- Ask colleagues to ask questions and to critique your presentation and answers.

(e) *Ready for the meeting.*
- Read and familiarize yourself with instructions issued by the meeting organizers to presenters.
- Confirm the time and place to hand in slide materials.
- Confirm the correct location of your presentation.
- Arrange to attend the presentation room ahead of time to view the controls and familiarize yourself with the layout.

## Presentation

Careful and timely preparation will allow you to approach your presentation with confidence and enthusiasm.

- **Talk** clearly, slowly and loudly but do not shout.
- **Face** and speak to the audience and not the screen.
- Be discreet with **pointers** or laser lights: overuse of pointers is distracting and you will lose the attention of the audience.
- **Microphone:** if using a stationary microphone, do talk towards it and avoid moving away. A clip-on microphone allows more freedom but a common mistake is to allow the microphone to continually rub your clothes as you move.
- **Timing** is essential during both preparation and presentation. Allow more time for your main points and less time for minor points. Finish within your allotted time, allowing time for questions. The impact of your conclusions will be lost if the chairperson is interrupting to ask you to finish.
- End your presentation clearly so the audience and chairperson know you are finished; for instance, perhaps thank the audience for taking the time to listen.

**Debrief**

After your presentation, note down your feelings as to what went well and what should be changed. Ask colleagues in the audience for their views. This will allow you to perform better next time.

## Further Reading

Davis M. *Scientific Papers and Presentations.* San Diego: Academic Press, 1997.
Turk C. *Effective speaking – communicating in speech.* London: Chapman & Hall, 1994.

## Related topics of interest

Audit, p. 188; Research process, p. 6.

# WRITING UP: CASE REPORTS, PUBLICATIONS AND THESIS

*Michael Kuo*

## Case reports and publications

**1. *Choice of journal.*** Choosing the journal to which one wishes to submit a paper brings many considerations.

(a) *The intended readers.* One of the considerations is the intended audience where there are overlapping specialty interests in the research study. For example, a paper on 'Preoperative cervical spine X-ray in children with Down syndrome undergoing general anaesthesia' may be appropriate for publication in a radiological, paediatric or anaesthetic journal. Bear in mind that 'dual publication,' where the same data are published in two or more papers, is unethical and will be censured.

(b) *Impact factor.* In scientific publications, an important consideration is the 'impact factor' or the 'Journal Citation Index' of the journal to which you wish to submit your paper. Its calculation is based on the number of times articles within the journal in question are cited in other peer-reviewed publications. Examples of the cited impact factors (1999) include: *Cell* 36.242, *Nature* 29.491, *Lancet* 10.197, *British Journal of Anaesthesia* 2.387 and *Journal of Neuro-ophthalmology* 0.374. The precise method of calculation of these factors and an up-to-date list is obtainable at http://wos.mimas.ac.uk . Clearly the choice of target journal requires ambition tempered by humility!

**2. *Technicalities.***

(a) *Instructions.* Having chosen the journal to which one is submitting a paper for review, the published instructions to authors should be read carefully.

- In some cases (like the *British Medical Journal*), these are only published in certain issues during the year, but most journals carry instructions to authors in the inside covers.
- There is no excuse for not adhering to style formats dictated by the journal. Should that occur, the best one could expect is a delay in review of the paper and at worst a quick rejection.
- Most journals expect a submission on hard copy as well as in an electronic format. One must ensure that an acceptable word-processing package is used.

(b) *Which section of the journal?* Most journals carry articles in well-defined sections, such as 'original papers', 'brief reports', 'radiology in focus', 'case reports', etc., and it is often helpful to state which section you wish your manuscript to be considered for.

**3. *Ethics.*** Ensure that an appropriate indication of ethical committee approval for the use of patient-related data is submitted to the journal. The consent of the patient is now required in case reports submitted to many journals.

**4. *Illustrations.*** The size of illustrations is usually determined by column width and must be closely adhered to. On the issue of illustrations, one should bear in mind the page costs which are sometimes payable for colour illustrations. Photographs should be kept to a minimum and only used to show important data or results.

**5. *Style.*** Each author has his/her particular style of presentation. However, it is often helpful to scan several recent issues of the journal being submitted to in order to gain a feel for the style of writing favoured by the journal's editors.

**6. *Authorship.*** Journals are increasingly questioning the role of individuals in the list of authors.

- This has arisen because of a tradition of 'gift authorship' for senior colleagues who have contributed little or nothing to the paper.
- It is essential that the contribution of each author listed can be identified and justified. Indeed, the *British Medical Journal* requires the nature of each author's involvement to be stated.
- The principal researcher should be the first author, with subsequent authors contributing progressively less to the paper with the exception of the final author, who is usually the senior researcher on the project. The first or senior author is usually also required to act as the guarantor of the paper, taking responsibility for the accuracy, originality and veracity of the data presented.
- It is important that all the authors sign the covering letter which accompanies the manuscript as failure to do this will result in delays in processing of the manuscript.

**7. *Summary.***
- One must choose the journal to which one is submitting a manuscript wisely, based on the appropriateness of the subject matter and a realistic evaluation of the likelihood of acceptance by that particular journal.
- Having done so, one must follow the instructions to the letter so that delays or rejections will not be due to typographical and technical shortcomings in the preparation of the manuscript.
- Finally, ensure that a well-crafted abstract succeeds in summarizing the aims and outcomes of the research as well as drawing the attention of the reviewer and subsequently the reader of your article.

## Thesis

The preparation of a thesis or dissertation is a considerable task. The key to the successful completion of a thesis lies in planning, preparation and scheduling.

**1. *Planning.***

(a) *Rules and regulations.*
- As with other publications, ensure that one is familiar with the rules and regulations before beginning to write a thesis.
- Each institution will have regulations regarding length of thesis (in words or pages), numbering of pages, style of referencing, width of margins, size of font and ordering of preliminary sections such as abstract, acknowledgements and contents tables.

- These are either published on the institution's web-site or printed copies may be available from the information services department.
- These considerations may appear mundane, but getting it right at the start saves a huge amount of time later on making corrections.

(b) *Reviewing others' theses.* Browsing through a number of theses from one's own department and collaborative departments is the ideal way of developing a framework for one's own thesis.

(c) *Initial ideas on layout.*
- From these precedents, one can establish a preference for format and style, for balance of topics and for presentation of illustrations, either on separate unnumbered pages or integrated into the main body of the text.
- The main advantage of integrating illustrations into the text is aesthetic and it is more convenient for the reader to refer from the text to a figure on the same page. However, the disadvantages are that there are limitations on the size of figures and addition or deletion of figures radically alters the page structures which often requires extensive realignment of paragraphs.

## 2. Preparation.

(a) *General introduction, material and methods.* It is wise and commonly given advice to write the general introduction early on in the research period and to update the introduction with time. Apart from consolidating one's grasp of the literature, having a substantial part of the thesis written when one starts on the results gives a large boost to the writing up process. The same advice can be applied to the topic on material and methods for similar reasons.

(b) *Literature review.* Central to the successful preparation of a thesis is an efficient and clear presentation of a comprehensive literature review. The cataloguing and subsequent presentation of one's literature review are immensely facilitated by the use of bibliographic software of which there are several available. The investment of time in learning how to use such software will be richly repaid if one is writing a case report and almost mandatory if one is planning to write a thesis. Bibliographic software options and use are covered in the topic 'Literature searching'; p. 11.

(c) *Develop computer skills.*
- While most people will be familiar with the use of a word-processor, writing a thesis may be the first time they use section and paragraph numbering extensively.
- All modern word-processors offer numbering functions, the principal advantages being that sections can be added or deleted without the need for manual renumbering and that a table of contents is automatically generated. It is useful to organize the numbering and the headings at the outset as it is often more difficult to do so later in the process. Therefore, seek advice on the use of these functions early on in the writing up process.

## 3. Scheduling. Scheduling is of great importance in the writing up of a thesis.

(a) *Communication between the student and the supervisor.* Central to the scheduling is good communication between the student and the supervisor. The supervisor should be able to recognize the point in the student's project at which a coherent thesis can be written and defended.

(b) *Prospectively agreed schedule.*
- A good hypothesis, when successfully examined, only yields more questions, and therefore in theory, a project is open-ended. Once the writing up process has started, the student should adhere to a prospectively agreed schedule and deliver appropriate 'aliquots' of the thesis for review and discussion with the supervisor.
- Robust scheduling is of particular importance to clinicians who are undertaking a period of full-time research in the context of a clinical training. The importance of completing the write-up of a thesis prior to returning to full-time clinical duties, for obvious reasons, can not be emphasized enough.

*4. Summary.* In summary, the preparation of a thesis is the culmination of a long period of intensive research. One should ensure that it is a coherent argument supported by an exhaustive bibliography. Remember that the defence of a meticulously presented thesis is invariably easier than the defence of one punctuated with inaccuracies.

## Further Reading

Cooter M. Putting on the style. *British Medical Journal* 1999; **319:** 1592.
Skelton JR, Edwards SJL. The function of the discussion section in academic medical writing. *British Medical Journal* 2000; **320:** 1269–1270.

## Related topics of interest

Laboratory research, p. 17; Literature searching, p. 11; Peer review, p. 185.

# REFERENCE MANAGEMENT

*Gavin D. Perkins*

The preparation and quotation of references are an integral part of writing a scientific paper or thesis. They provide a mechanism which enables the work of others to be recognized and acknowledged and to support statements made in the text of a paper. They also allow the reader to identify and retrieve the sources of information quoted, quickly and easily.

## Preparation

When preparing a manuscript and reference list it is important to check the precise details that are required by the organization or publisher. Many journals have minor variations on the established referencing systems (such as when to use *italics* and **bold**) so the precise description on how to format references should be checked on each occasion. For medical journals this information can be found in the Guide to Contributors of the journal. Whilst the full Guide to Contributors is rarely published in every edition of a journal, details of where the information can be found are usually included. This information is also available in many instances on the journal's website.

A variety of different systems exist for presenting references in the text of medical journals and theses. The principal systems in use today are the Vancouver and Harvard systems. The Vancouver system is the format required by most biomedical journals, whilst the Harvard system is used predominantly by biological, social science and education journals.

## Vancouver system

This system assigns consecutive numbers to identify references as they occur in the text. A reference list is then prepared at the end of the paper or topic in numerical order.

***1. Example.*** Ashbaugh and colleagues[1] first described the condition that is now known as the acute respiratory distress syndrome over thirty years ago. Since these early descriptions, a number of groups have refined the diagnostic criteria for this condition[2-4]. Some journals use numbers in square brackets (e.g. [2–4]) instead of superscript numerals.

*References*
1. Ashbaugh DG, Bigelow DB, Petty TL, Levine BE. Acute respiratory distress in adults. *Lancet* 1967; **2**: 319–323.
2. Petty TL, Ashbaugh DG. The adult respiratory distress syndrome: clinical features, factors influencing prognosis and principles of management. *Chest* 1971; **60**: 233–239.
3. Murray JF, Matthay MA, Luce JM, Flick MR. An expanded definition of the adult respiratory distress syndrome. *Am Rev Respir Dis* 1988; **138**: 720–723.
4. Bernard GR, Artigas A, Brigham KL, Carlet J, Falke K, Hudson L et al. The American-European Consensus Conference on ARDS: definitions, mechanisms, relevant outcomes, and clinical trial coordination. *Am J Respir Crit Care Med* 1994; **149**: 818–824.

**2. Formats.** Depending on the source of the material (journal, book topic, on-line reference etc), different formats can apply to the construction of references in the reference list.

*(a)* Article from a journal
- Individual authors. Author(s) initial(s). Title of the article. *Title of the journal* year of publication; **Volume**: first–last page numbers. E.g. Chopra V, Gesink BJ, De Jong J, Bovill JG, Spierdijk J, Brand R. Does training on an anaesthesia simulator lead to improvement in performance? *Br J Anaesth* 1994; **73**: 293–297.
- Organization as an author. E.g. Royal College of Physicians (London). Resuscitation from cardiopulmonary arrest. Training and organisation. A report of the Royal College of Physicians. J R Coll Physicians Lond 1987; 21: 175–182.
- No author. E.g. Insights into Pulmonary Embolism [editorial]. *BMJ* 1991; **84**: 15.
- Notes:
    1. More than 6 authors – List first 6 authors followed by *et al.*
    2. Issue number and month of publication are required by some journals in which case they are included in brackets after the volume number, e.g. Br J Anaesth 1994; 73(2): 293–297.
    3. Standard abbreviations for journals (listed in *Index Medicus*) should be used. This list can also be obtained from the US National Library of Medicine (http://www.nlm.nih.gov/).

(b) *Books*
- Entire book written by one or more authors. Author(s) initial(s). *Title of book*. Edition number. Place of publication: Publisher; Date of publication. E.g. Ryder REJ, Mir MA, Freeman EA. *An Aid to the MRCP Short Cases*. 1st ed. London: Blackwell-Scientific; 1986.
- Entire book quoting editors as authors. Author(s) initial(s), editors. *Title of book*. Edition. Place of publication: Publisher, Date of publication. E.g. Greaves I, Hodgetts T, Porter K, editors. *Emergency Care: A textbook for Paramedics*. 1st ed. London: W.B. Saunders, 1997.
- Topic in a book. Topic author Surname(s) initial(s). Title of the topic. In: Editors Surname(s) initial(s) editors. *Title of the book*. Edition. Place of publication: Publisher; Date of publication. p. page numbers. E.g. Bion JF. Severity and outcomes of critical illness. In: Oh TE, editor. *Intensive Care Medicine*. 4th ed. Bath (UK): Butterworth-Heinemann; 1987. p. 11–16.
- Organization as author and publisher. E.g. Resuscitation Council (UK). Advanced Life Support Course. 4th ed. London: Resuscitation Council UK; 2000.

(c) Dissertation. E.g. Barton AE. A study of factors influencing the destructive potential of human neutrophils. [Ph.D thesis]. University of Birmingham; 1996.

(d) Electronic citations. Morse SS. Factors in the emergence of infectious diseases. Emerg Infect Dis [serial online] 1995 Jan–Mar [cited 1996 Jun 5]; 1(1):[24 screens]. Available from: URL: http://www.cdc.gov/ncidod/EID/eid.htm

### 3. Other formats

(a) Articles in supplements. Supplement number follows volume number. e.g. '**105 Suppl 1**: 277–289'.

(b) Personal communication. Avoid this whenever possible. If it is essential, it should be included in the text as [Gao F, personal communication] but not appear in the reference list. Written confirmation that it is acceptable to quote the individual in this format should ideally be sought.

(c) In press. Articles in press should be identified as such, e.g. Tweed MJ, Miola J. Legal Challenge. *Medical Teacher* 2001; In press.

The description for formatting other less frequently cited sources can be found in 'Uniform Requirements for Manuscripts submitted to Biomedical Journals'.

## Harvard System

The Harvard system uses author and date of publication in the text to cite a reference. The list of references at the end of the work is arranged alphabetically by author's surname and year of publication.

> **1. *Example.*** Ashbaugh and others (1967) first described the condition that is now known as the acute respiratory distress syndrome. Since these early descriptions a number of groups have refined the diagnostic criteria for this condition. (Bernard et al. 1994; Murray et al. 1988; Petty & Ashbaugh 1971).

*References*
Ashbaugh, D. G., Bigelow, D. B., Petty, T. L., & Levine, B. E. (1967). "Acute respiratory distress in adults". *Lancet*, **2**, 319–323
Bernard, G. R., Artigas, A., Brigham, K. L., Carlet, J., Falke, K., Hudson, L., Lamy, M., Legall, J. R., Morris, A., & Spragg, R. (1994). "The American-European Consensus Conference on ARDS. Definitions, mechanisms, relevant outcomes, and clinical trial coordination". *Am.J.Respir.Crit. Care Med*, **149** (3 Pt 1), 818–824.
Murray, J. F., Matthay, M. A., Luce, J. M., & Flick, M. R. (1988). "An expanded definition of the adult respiratory distress syndrome". *Am.Rev.Respir.Dis.*, **138**, 720–723.
Petty, T. L. & Ashbaugh, D. G. (1971). "The adult respiratory distress syndrome. Clinical features, factors influencing prognosis and principles of management". *Chest*, **60**, 233–239.

### 2. Notes.

(a) When the author's name occurs naturally in the sentence then the date of the reference only is required (i.e. no need for duplication of the surname). e.g. Ashbaugh and others (1967).

(b) When the author's name is not included as part of the sentence then the author's surname and the year the work was published are inserted in the text to cite the reference. Up to two authors may be included in the text citation, e.g. (Petty & Ashbaugh 1971).

(c) When more than two authors are listed for a paper then the text citation is changed to the first author's name followed by 'et al.' or 'and others', e.g. (Bernard *et al.* 1994).

(d) As described above, the reference list is then arranged in alphabetical order according to the first author's surname.

(e) If there is more than one reference by the same author, they are arranged chronologically, with the earlier publication date first.

(f) If the same author has written several articles in the same year they are differentiated by the lower case letters a,b,c,d etc., following the date in the text and the reference list.

E.g. 'Matthay (2002a) recently reviewed....... Novel strategies for enhancing alveolar fluid clearance......(Matthay *et al.*, 2002b).

Matthay, M. A. (2002a) "Regulation of ion and fluid transport across the distal pulmonary epithelia: new insights", *Am.J.Physiol Lung Cell Mol.Physiol.* **282 (4)**, L595–L598.

Matthay, M. A., Uchida, T., & Fang, X. (2002b) "Clinical Acute Lung Injury and Acute Respiratory Distress Syndrome". *Current treatment options in cardiovascular medicine* **4 (2)**, 139–149.

## Reference storage and retrieval

It is very important to develop a system for methodically recording reference details. A little time spent setting up a system during the background reading phase of a research project will save a great deal of time when it comes to the writing phase later on. The development of computer-based reference management software has revolutionized the storage and retrieval of references. In the past, authors would spend hours/days developing handwritten or word-processed reference lists. Using these software packages, it is now possible to download references from Internet-based bibliographic databases such as Medline and the Web of Science and store them directly in your own database of references. In addition to the standard reference details (author names, title, paper, page numbers, etc.), abstracts, keywords and web addresses (if available) may also be downloaded and stored. Alternatively, references may be entered manually or downloaded from other sources such as CD-Rom based bibliographic databases.

The software packages are compatible with most word-processing packages. This allows references to be inserted into the text of a document and a reference list generated at the click of a button, saving many hours of time manually typing them in. The packages can automatically re-number the reference list if the order of references is changed during editing. The user can often specify the style of the references in the reference list. This could either be an empirical format such as the Vancouver or Harvard system described above, or in the specific format required by a particular medical journal.

There are several software packages available on the market and include: Papyrus, Procite, Endnote and Reference Manager. It is important to check the software's compatibility with your chosen word-processing package and to ensure that it will allow the input and output of data in a flexible form before purchasing.

## Further reading

Halsey MJ. References. In: Hall GM (ed). *How to write a paper.* 1st edition. London: BMJ Publishing; 1994, p 42–51.

Information Services. *Preparing and Quoting References.* Birmingham(UK):University of Birmingham; 2001. Also available from http://www.is.bham.ac.uk/publications/skills/preparing.pdf (accessed 23-10-2001).

Uniform Requirements for Manuscripts Submitted to Biomedical Journals. *Journal of the American Medical Association* 1997; **277:** 927–934. Also available from
http://jama.ama-assn.org/info/auinst_req.html (accessed 23-10-2001).

## Related topics of interest

Literature searching, p. 11; Research process, p. 6; Writing up: case report, publications and thesis, p. 176.

# PEER REVIEW

*Michael Vickers*

Editors cannot hope to be expert on every topic submitted for publication. They therefore maintain a panel of experts to guide them. They usually select two (sometimes three) whom they believe can provide an expert opinion on your paper. This is known as 'Peer Review,' implying that you and they are equally expert. The editor may pass on the comments of these referees as a *précis* or verbatim: either way, the author(s) must respond appropriately.

## Purpose of using expert referees

To ensure that your paper can be relied on, it must be:

- Scientifically valid;
- Its conclusions justified.

It is essentially a paternalistic process, assuming that the readers are insufficiently expert to make these decisions. When the readers are likely to all be expert this is less important. Some journals already publish unrefereed material on the Internet.

## Functions of the referee

A good review will start with a summary of what the paper is about: basically a *précis* of your abstract. It will offer comments on some or all of the following aspects, as appropriate:

- The originality of the idea behind the study;
- The importance of the work for other researchers;
- The likely benefit to patients;
- Readability and presentation;
- Errors and ambiguities;
- Queries on the method;
- Queries on the statistics;
- Whether your conclusions are justified;
- Specific criticisms and suggested amendments.

The editor reserves the right to decide on acceptance but may request the referees' opinion.

## The editor's letter

Read this carefully: apart from any specific points raised by the referees, it will contain phraseology on a continuum which will guide your response, ranging through:

(a) I am happy to publish your paper ($+/-$ with minor editorial amendments).
(b) I will publish your paper if you can make the changes suggested.
(c) Please respond to the referees' comments ($+/-$ and submit a revised manuscript).
(d) In view of the referees' comments I cannot accept this for publication in its present form.

(e) In view of the referees' comments I am unable to accept your paper for publication.

Response (a) calls for no action: response (e) is so discouraging that a response may be a waste of time, although it depends on what they have actually said. Responses (b, c & d) call for action.

## Answering the editor/referees

Do not lose your temper at what may appear to be unfounded criticisms. Your reply must be thoughtful and thorough. If not already done, number each point. Analyse the points under three headings: simple misunderstandings, typographical errors, etc., criticisms which can be met and criticisms to which there is no answer.

1. *Simple misunderstandings.* These should be easy to deal with.

2. *Criticisms which can be met by amendments.*

- Of the method: have you given enough detail?
- Of the statistics: a job for an expert. Most common is failing to calculate the power of the study.
- Of the conclusions: usually going beyond the evidence. Make sure you have included a paragraph on analysing why your results might be suspect.
- Of the references: have you quoted selectively from papers which support your conclusions?

3. *Criticisms which cannot be met by amendments.*

- Having too small a sample for the conclusions: you cannot just extend the trial, having broken the code.
- Flawed method or inappropriate use: you must convince the editor that this is not true. You must be more 'expert' than his experts!
- Incorrect trial design: too late now – but it may be the correct design for a slightly different question and different conclusions.

## Editorial criticisms

If the editor requests that your paper be shortened, there are at least five possible causes which you can remedy:

(a) You have written a mini-thesis which contains a lot of background material which is well established, uncontentious and known to all relevant readers.
(b) You have repeated much of your introduction at the start of your discussion.
(c) You have tried to discuss too many points arising from the results: reduce to between three to five.
(d) The same data are given in both tables and figures or repeated *in extenso* in the text.
(e) There is unjustified extrapolation or speculation in the discussion.

## Your reply

This consists of a covering letter to the editor, a detailed response to each point raised by either referee and, if indicated, a revised manuscript.

1. *Covering letter.* Express gratitude for the helpful comments, which have all been dealt with and which have improved the paper. Enclosed is a revised script in

which all the changes have been highlighted to assist him. Do not disparage the referees' expertise: any lapse on their part is due to misunderstandings to which you have no doubt contributed!

**2. *Detailed response.*** This needs as much work and care as the original paper. All authors must be involved in the response. Unless previously consulted, a statistician may need to be recruited to your cause. Use each numbered criticism as a paragraph heading of your response. Your 'tone' must be neutral and scientific. Your aim is to show that you are indeed the more expert.

**3. *Revised manuscript.*** As well as a script showing the changes, submit the required number of unmarked copies.

## If the paper is rejected

Can the paper be resuscitated? If so, it can be re-submitted to the same journal or sent to another one.

If any major criticism is made which cannot be answered but which appears misguided, you can appeal to the editor for a review. To succeed, such an appeal requires cogent arguments. If you believe that despite its rejection you can eventually meet the criticisms adequately, signal your intention to re-submit in your response to the editor's letter.

If you decide to submit elsewhere it is essential to deal as fully as possible with the criticisms in a revised manuscript. Remember, many referees act for more than one journal. To limit this risk, one can submit to a journal published in another country or to a 'rival' journal in the same country. It can be quite disarming to tell the new editor the full story: if you can persuade a senior and respected colleague to assist with the revision – or at least check it, do not forget to acknowledge this help. Apart from professional courtesy, it may reassure the editor that such a person has been prepared to see his or her name associated with the paper.

## Further reading

Vickers MD. How to get published: the peer review process. In: Zbinden AM, Thomson D (eds) *Conducting Research in Anaesthesia and Intensive Care Medicine.* Oxford: Butterworth Heinemann, 2001, pp. 266–277.

## Related topic of interest

Writing up: case reports, publications and thesis, p. 176.

# AUDIT

*Danny McAuley*

Audit is a process by which health professionals assess, evaluate and improve health care. Audit is not a new concept and extends as far back as Hippocrates who reported on the outcome of the patients he treated. Healthcare professionals have been undertaking audit for many years, although more recently this process has been formalized. Audit is frequently undertaken as part of quality assessment and quality assurance programmes.

## Definitions

**1. Audit.** The Department of Health White Paper 'Working for Patients' defined audit as 'the systematic, critical analysis of the quality of medical care, including the procedures used for diagnosis and treatment, the use of resources, and the resulting outcome and quality of life for the patient.'

**2. Quality assessment and assurance.** Quality assessment involves determining the extent to which current care achieves predetermined standards. Quality assurance is the process undertaken in the light of any deficiencies in care identified through quality assessment.

**3. Medical and clinical audit.** Medical audit refers to audit undertaken by medical staff, while clinical audit refers to audit undertaken by any group of healthcare professionals.

## Types of audit

Audit may relate to three aspects:

**1. Structure.** Audit of structure assesses the quality of the environment in which care is provided (e.g., working hours).

**2. Process.** Audit of process assesses the quality of care delivered (e.g., blood transfusion protocol).

**3. Outcome.** Audit of outcome assesses patient benefit (e.g., postoperative pain relief, postoperative morbidity and mortality).

It is possible for an audit to address all three aspects of healthcare delivery.

## The audit cycle

The audit cycle is made up of six stages:

1. *Define criteria and standards* for the matter of interest.
2. *Collect data* on current performance.
3. *Assess extent to which current practice achieves criteria and standards.*
4. *Identify areas* in which current practice may be improved.
5. *Implement change.*
6. *Re-audit* after the planned changes have been implemented.

## Who undertakes audit

Audit may be undertaken by:

1. *An individual* as part of the process of self-audit.
2. *A colleague*, who is of the same standing, an equal, as part of peer-audit.
3. *An external group* as part of external audit.

These different forms of audit are not mutually exclusive and may be undertaken in combination.

## Designing an audit project

If it is to be of any benefit, consideration must be given to the design of the project prior to undertaking an audit. Healthcare trainees are frequently under pressure to undertake an audit project to fulfil a requirement of their training. As a result, many audits are undertaken with little thought for design and provide little or no improvement in patient care.

An audit project should:

- be relevant and important to those undertaking the audit;
- have the potential to improve healthcare delivery;
- have attainable aims within the resources available;
- address a clearly defined question;
- have a plan data for collection which is viable and which will provide an answer to the question being asked.

**1.  *Defining criteria and standards for area of interest.*** The expected standard of care must be defined prior to undertaking an audit project.

(a) *Criterion and standard*
- A criterion is used to describe a definable aspect of health care and a standard refers to the acceptable level of care for a particular criterion.
- The statement that patients with cardiac failure should receive an angiotensin converting enzyme (ACE) inhibitor is a criterion and the statement that 80% of patients with cardiac failure should receive an ACE inhibitor is a standard.
- There is a potential disadvantage with explicit measurable statements in that there will be a tendency to focus only on what can be measured.

(b) *Basis of criteria and standards*
- Criteria and standards should be based on best available clinical evidence or, in the absence of evidence, expert consensus opinion.
- Standards should be clear and focused on the proposed audit. Unfortunately, many audits are undertaken without clearly defined *a priori* standards and, as a result, can become exercises in data collection which do not address any specific question.

**2.  *Data collection.*** Data collection may be prospective or retrospective.

(a) *Prospective*
- Data are collected forwards in time from the start of the audit to provide information on the current or subsequent practice.

- Prospective data should be more accurate than retrospective data and may thereby minimise bias.
- However, healthcare professionals may consciously or unconsciously alter their practice if they are aware that a prospective audit is taking place.

(b) *Retrospective*
- Data are collected backwards in time from the start of the audit to provide information on past practice.
- Data are often collected from medical records, or a clinical computing database or by interview.
- However, medical records have major limitations in that the information contained in them may be incomplete or even inaccurate. This represents an important source of bias.

### 3. Data analysis.

(a) *Aims*
- To compare performance with predetermined standards;
- to identify areas for improvement; and
- to develop methods which can be implemented to improve health care.

(b) *Screening the data*
- A considerable amount of data can be generated by audit even when only a small number of cases are being examined.
- When large amounts of data are collected it is possible that a previously unrecognised aspect of healthcare may be identified.
- More commonly, large amounts of irrelevant data make interpretation difficult or even meaningless and the key aim of the audit is lost. Only relevant data that answer the primary audit questions should be analyzed.

(c) *Statistical analysis*
- The purpose of using statistical analysis in an audit study is to identify the difference between the performance and predetermined standards.
- Descriptive statistics and appropriate comparison statistics are usually adequate.

### 4. Presentation.
Keep the presentation as simple as possible. The structure of a presentation should include:

- *Objectives.*
- *Defining set of standards.*
- *Methods:* data collection and analysis.
- *Results:* it can be difficult to extract data from tables which summarize many facts. Graphical presentation of data provides much more effective communication of information.
- *Conclusions* and plan for a re-audit.

## Audit or research

### 1. Similarities.

(a) *Types of clinical audit studies*
Clinical research may be broadly classified as experimental studies or observational studies (see 'Research design', p. 31). Clinical audit studies resemble clinical observational studies as shown in *Figure 1*.

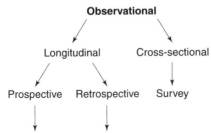

Figure 1. Types of clinical audit studies.

(b) *Conduct of an audit study*
As in research, an audit study involves the establishment of an idea, the design of the project, the collection and analysis of data, presentation and publication.

### 2. Differences.

*Objectives of the process.*
Audit aims to improve healthcare by comparison against a standard. By contrast, the aim of research is to test a hypothesis and may include the objective of defining best practice. This may be an arbitrary definition as, clearly, research can be undertaken in the context of routine clinical practice.

### 3. Ethical issues.

- Small locally organized audits may not need ethical approval and individual patient consent.

- However, the status of large-scale audits designed to influence broader practice remains unclear. Guidelines published by the Royal College of Physicians suggest submission to a LREC if doubt exists about whether a project is audit or research.

- It is desirable to submit an audit study to the LREC if the study is planned to be published

## Limitations of audit

Audit has limitations.

**1. Inappropriate subject.** It is inappropriate to audit an area where care is known to be excellent, but avoid audit in an area where there is a concern.

**2. *Misinterpretation of the aim of audit.*** Audit can be threatening and it is important to emphasize that audit is undertaken to improve health care and not to identify responsibility for poor care.

**3. *Person performing audit.*** With peer-review audit, deficiencies in the provision of health care which are common to both the peer (person undertaking audit) and the person being audited may result in failure to recognize such deficiencies. Although external audit has the theoretical advantage of greater objectivity, such audit can be more threatening.

**4. *Failures in improvement.*** Audit frequently fails to bring about the planned change and improvement in health care. Although in theory the audit cycle should lead to improvement in health care, there are complex reasons why this does not occur. In many cases, audit is undertaken merely to show that the relevant health professionals can be seen to be doing it, regardless of outcome. Until a greater priority is placed upon audit, it is unlikely that appropriately designed audit studies, able to generate meaningful results that can be acted upon, and with adequate funding to implement change, will be undertaken. Until this occurs audit is unlikely to produce significant healthcare improvement.

## Further reading

Guidelines for developing an audit project. *The Royal College of Anaesthetists Bulletin* 2001; **8:** 375.

Irvine D, Irvine S. *Making Sense of Audit.* Oxford: Radcliffe Medical Press, 1991.

Johnston G, Crombie IK, Alder EM, Davies HTO, Millard A. Reviewing audit: barriers and facilitating factors for effective clinical audit. *Quality in Health Care* 2000; **9:** 23–36.

Lord J, Littlejohns P. Evaluating healthcare policies: the case of clinical audit. *British Medical Journal* 1997; **315:** 668–671.

## Related topics of interest

Research process, p. 6; Research design, p. 31; ICNARC, p. 196.

# RISK ADJUSTMENT AND STANDARDIZED MORTALITY RATIO

*Liam Lynch*

## Risk adjustment

This is the process by which outcomes (usually mortality) in health care are evaluated against the severity of illness in the patient population being studied. In the United Kingdom, risk adjustment is most developed in Intensive Care and Accident & Emergency medicine. Worldwide, risk adjustment has also been used in containing healthcare costs, in evaluating coronary artery surgery and for improving quality in healthcare systems.

## Risk adjustment methods

***1. Acute physiology and chronic health evaluation (APACHE).*** This method of risk adjustment is used in intensive care medicine and is a severity of illness scoring system.

(a) *Methodology.*
- These systems are produced by prospective data collection on large numbers of patients.
- Regression analysis is then used to identify and weigh various patient factors which are important predictors of outcome.
- An equation of risk adjustment may then be produced.

(b) *The APACHE II score.*
- The APACHE II score includes 12 physiological variables, patient age and chronic health conditions.
- This score, in combination with a diagnostic category, can generate an expected mortality for the patient.
- The APACHE II system has been updated to APACHE III but this is a commercial product and the resulting equation is not in the public domain. Whilst APACHE III scores may be calculated, they are not useful in risk adjustment without the equation.

***2. The trauma injury severity score (TRISS).*** This system is used in a similar way in accident & emergency medicine.

- The human body is divided into six areas and injuries to each area scored from 1 to 5. For example, a bruised upper limb would score 1 point and a traumatic amputation 5 points.
- The scores for the three worst affected areas are squared to produce a final result between 3 and 75, which again may be used to calculate the risk of death.

***3. New York Heart Association (NYHA) score.*** This groups patients with cardiac disease into categories by functional definitions. Outcomes after cardiac surgery may then be interpreted in the light of the patient population distribution through each category.

**4. _The Goldman cardiac risk index._** This is used in anaesthesia to score patients with ischaemic heart disease who present for non-cardiac surgery. The score may indicate which patients are at highest risk.

## Validation of risk adjustment methods

Risk adjustment methods should be validated independently against a new population. There are two tests commonly used for validation.

**1. _Calibration test._** This examines the extent of the agreement between the expected and actual numbers of hospital deaths in a new population. The expected number of hospital deaths is compared with the actual number of deaths and this agreement can be tested formally using a goodness-of-fit statistic.

**2. _Discrimination test._** This examines the ability of a risk adjustment method to determine patients who live from patients who die, based on the expected hospital deaths. This process generates a receiver operating characteristic (ROC) curve. The greater the true positive rate (the proportion of patients predicted to die who actually die) relative to the false-positive rate (the proportion of patients predicted to die who live), the greater the area under the ROC curve. The area under the curve should be at least 80% if the method is valid.

## Uses of risk adjustment methods

Risk adjustment methods may have two main uses:

- To compare different units and hospitals in their death rates either using individual actual mortality compared with the average actual mortality of units or hospitals or using standardized mortality ratios;
- To stratify patients in randomized controlled trials, multi-centre trials or audit studies.

## Limitations of risk adjustment methods

- Results are affected by inaccurate data collection following lack of standardized variables, such as the primary reason for ICU admission, or by missing data.
- Results are affected by 'lead-time bias' that is caused by different treatments of a patient, e.g. stabilized or untreated, before admission to intensive care.
- Results may be affected by an intervention, e.g. altering heart rate.
- Different risk adjustment methods estimate different expected hospital death rates for the same cohort of patients. Therefore, it is inappropriate to use a risk adjustment method as the basis for clinical decision-making in individual patients.

## Standardized mortality ratio (SMR)

SMR is the ratio of _the actual_ mortality rate to the _expected_ mortality rate in a population group. Values of <1.0 indicate a better than expected outcome. Conversely, values >1.0 indicate a poorer than expected outcome.

Confidence intervals can be calculated to determine if the difference from 1.0 is statistically significant.

The expected death rate may be derived from population studies, historical data or scoring systems such as APACHE II.

**1. SMR obtained from population study.** If we assume that the death rate nationally from road traffic accidents is 12 per 100 000 of the population per annum, then the safety or otherwise of a given area may be compared to this rate. If in Dorset for example the rate was 15 per 100 000 per annum, then the SMR would be 1.25 – indicating a higher than average death rate. However, this does not tell the whole story as there may be a great deal of variability in the rates across the country and the Dorset rate may be within normal limits. More information is therefore required to calculate the confidence intervals of national traffic death rates.

**2. SMR obtained from a scoring system.** In intensive care medicine all patients who qualify for APACHE II scoring will generate an expected mortality of between 0 and 1. The sum of these expected mortalities for an individual unit is then the expected number of deaths prior to hospital discharge. This is compared to the actual death rate and an SMR produced. In the UK the overall SMRs produced using the APACHE II system are consistently above 1 and this has given rise to a great deal of debate, but no conclusion as yet.

## Further reading

Intensive Care National Audit and Research centre. Annual report from the case mix programme dataset. 2001; p. 31.
Rowan K. Risk adjustment for intensive care outcomes. In: Goldhill DR, Withington PS (eds). *Textbook of Intensive Care*. London, Chapman & Hall Medical, 1997.

## Related topics of interest

# INTENSIVE CARE NATIONAL AUDIT AND RESEARCH CENTRE (ICNARC)

*Liam Lynch*

ICNARC is a charity whose function is to initiate and undertake audit and research projects in association with intensive care units in the United Kingdom. It was founded in 1994 and is based in London.

Dr Kathy Rowan the director and founder of ICNARC co-ordinated the Intensive Care Society's UK Acute Physiology And Chronic Health Evaluation (APACHE) II Study in 1988–90, published in 1993, which formed the basis of her Ph.D thesis. As a result of this study she wrote a proposal on behalf of the Society to establish an Audit and Research Centre. 'Pump-priming' funds were granted for 2 years by the Department of Health and the Welsh Health Common Services Authority. The Centre was established in 1994 and began recruiting units to the national audit in 1995. The Centre is now funded by the subscriptions of units participating in the national audit, by research grants and by consultancy fees.

At this time, there are two main areas of activity – audit (a national comparative audit called the Case Mix Programme) and research.

## Case Mix Programme

- All of ICNARC's participating intensive care units collect detailed data on every patient admitted. These include demographic, physiological, diagnostic and outcome data. The physiological data are based on the patient's first 24 hours in the unit and include all the data required for the commonly used scoring systems such as APACHE II, III, Simplified Acute Physiology Score (SAPS) II and Mortality Prediction Models (MPM) II. Paediatric Risk of Mortality (PRISM) data are also collected for paediatric admissions (*Figures 1* and *2*).

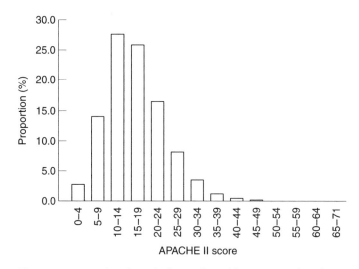

Figure 1. Example of analysis produced by ICNARC for the Case Mix Programme: distribution of APACHE II score.

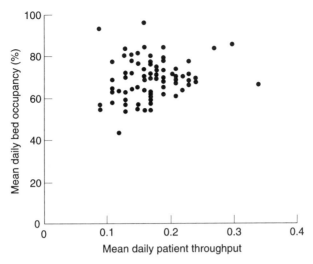

Figure 2. Example of analysis produced by ICNARC for the Case Mix Programme: bed occupancy versus patient throughput by unit. Note: units at the top right-hand corner have high occupancy and throughput – they are the busiest.

- ICNARC has developed its own hierarchical diagnostic coding method, which is based on the admission type (surgical/non-surgical), the body system, the anatomical site, the physiological/pathological disease process and the condition. For example, a patient with pneumonia would be coded as medical, respiratory, lungs, infection, and bacterial pneumonia. This generates a five-digit code. Over seven hundred codes, relating to various diagnoses are available. Underlying conditions rather than events (cardiac arrest) or procedures (tracheostomy) are coded.
- Each intensive care unit, involved in the Programme, submits their data to ICNARC on a 6-monthly basis. The data are then checked and may require several revisions before being validated. The initial submission generates a data validation report (DVR) on which incomplete data, grossly abnormal data and inconsistent data are queried. These are then checked locally. In some cases, several DVRs may be required before the data are completely validated. Upon completion of data validation, ICNARC issues a comparative data analysis report.
- The report summarizes the *individual* intensive care unit's data and compares them with the collective data within the Case Mix Programme Database. As of March 2001, ICNARC had received data on over 140,000 admissions, of which over 87,000 had been validated.
- Individual admissions/units/hospitals are not identified by ICNARC. The source of data is absolutely confidential and this is covered by a legal agreement between ICNARC and the participating unit/hospital.
- A recent (May 2000) policy document from the Department of Health (Comprehensive Critical Care) recommended that all adult, general intensive

care units should participate in the Case Mix Programme and that data collection should be an integral part of the provision of intensive care. Presently, more than 70% of adult, general intensive care units in England participate (64% Northern Ireland, 56% Wales). The West Midlands, North West and Eastern regions of the NHS have reached 100% participation. However, participation is lowest in London and South East regions.

- The benefits of participation in the Case Mix Programme include the availability of high-quality data for risk-adjusted outcome comparisons, for developing research projects and answering research questions. In addition, the network of participating units forms a source of committed intensive care units for collaboration in multicentre research studies.

## Research

- ICNARC co-ordinates and conducts multicentre research projects of relevance to intensive care in the UK. It focuses on both methodological and evaluative research projects.
- An early research project conducted by ICNARC generated a database of randomized controlled trials from hand-searching the intensive care and emergency medicine literature. The results of this work formed an important contribution to the Cochrane Collaboration.
- Current research projects include: using consensus methods to establish research priorities in intensive care medicine; assessing the optimum method for risk adjustment in both adult and paediatric intensive care; and a survey of attitudes to safety and teamwork in the intensive care unit. In addition, ICNARC is co-ordinating a large multicentre, randomized controlled trial of the clinical and cost-effectiveness of the pulmonary artery catheter (the PAC-Man Study). Over 70 intensive care units are participating in the PAC-Man Study and intensive care, as a speciality, has been praised for its ability to perform such a trial of an accepted intervention.
- Some of the research projects form the basis of doctoral theses for individual staff members and associated clinicians.
- During the year 2000, ICNARC was directly involved in 15 publications in the medical literature – ranging from results of primary research projects to results of secondary research – a systematic review of outcome measures in intensive care.
- More information about ICNARC and its work can be obtained by visiting www.icnarc.org.

## Acknowledgement

I am indebted to Dr. Kathy Rowan of ICNARC for her assistance with the preparation of this topic.

# Further reading

Angus D, Black N. Wider lessons of the pulmonary artery catheter trial. Intensivists are rising to the challenge of evaluating established practices. *British Medical Journal* 2001; **322**: 446.

Black NA, Jenkinson C, Hayes JA, Young JD, Vella K, Rowan KM, Daly K, Ridley S. A review of outcome measures used in adult critical care. *Critical Care Medicine*, 2001; **29**: 2119–2124.

Goldfrad C, Rowan K. Consequences of discharges from intensive care at night. *Lancet* 2000; **355:** 1138–1142.

Goldfrad C, Vella K, Bion J, Rowan K, Black N. Research priorities in critical care medicine in the UK. *Intensive Care Medicine* 2000; **26:** 1480–1488.

Langham J, Thompson E, Rowan K. Identification of randomised controlled trials from the emergency medicine literature: comparison of hand searching versus MEDLINE searching. *Annals of Emergency Medicine* 1999; **34:** 25–34.

Rowan KM, Black N. A bottom-up approach to performance indicators through clinician networks. Health Care UK, Spring 2000: 43–46.

Vella K, Goldfrad C, Rowan K, Bion JF, Black NA. Use of consensus development to establish national research priorities in critical care. *British Medical Journal* 2000; **320:** 976–980.

Young JD, Goldfrad C, Rowan K (on behalf of the ICNARC Coding Method Working Group). Development and testing of a hierarchical method to code the reason for admission to intensive care units: the ICNARC Coding Method. *British Journal of Anaesthesia* 2001; **87:** 543–548.

## Related topics of interest

Audit, p. 188; Risk adjustment and standardized mortality ratio, p. 193; Survival data, p. 155.

# PROTOCOLS AND GUIDELINES

*Liam Lynch*

Protocols and guidelines are to be found everywhere in modern life. From the diplomatic world to the smallest hospital they are an integral part of society. State funerals, for example, use a rigid protocol to decide who sits where and who is part of the cortege.

## Definitions

*1.* **Protocol.** A clinical protocol is an established set of rules governing the management of a particular clinical situation. In general terms, a protocol is best used in a situation which has a limited number of variables and the potential to achieve a 'correct' result.

*2.* **Guideline.** A guideline is an official recommendation guiding or directing a clinical activity. Generally, a guideline is best used where there are many variables and the outcome is less certain. A protocol is more rigid with little or no place for deviation, whereas a guideline allows for more variation.

## Clinical protocols and guidelines

In medicine, the best-known protocols are probably those associated with the Advanced Life Support programme. For cardiac arrest there are only a few possible electrical phenomena – asystole, ventricular fibrillation/tachycardia and pulseless electrical activity. A rigid protocol is therefore appropriate. However, in many medical situations there are far more potential problems and a guideline is a better solution. For instance, the British Thoracic Society has issued guidelines on the antibiotic management of community-acquired pneumonia but these may need to be modified in the light of local microbial resistance patterns.

## Development of clinical protocols and guidelines

Protocols or guidelines may be developed locally, regionally, nationally or internationally.

- They should meet a real need and be useful in clinical practice;
- For national guidelines, a working party may be formed comprising recognized experts in the field, for example, those who have published widely in the area concerned. Local guidelines may well be developed by an individual or a small group;
- They should be evidence-based (grading of evidence and recommendations are discussed below);
- Where national protocols or guidelines exist there is little point in re-inventing them locally;
- They should be easily understood and well laid out;
- They should be readily available;
- All staff must be aware of the protocol or guideline's existence;
- All staff should have regular updates on the protocol or the guideline;
- Compliance with the protocol or the guideline should be audited regularly;

- In some cases, e.g. Major Accident Plans, it may be appropriate to run test scenarios;
- They should be reviewed or updated at pre-determined intervals – usually from one to three years;
- For local protocols or guidelines a designated individual should be responsible for all of the above.

### Grading of evidence

The US Agency for Health Care Policy and Research suggests the following levels of evidence:

- Systematic reviews and meta-analyses of randomized controlled trials;
- Randomized controlled trials;
- Non-randomized intervention studies;
- Observational studies;
- Non-experimental studies;
- Expert opinion.

These levels have been expanded by Harbour & Miller (see Further reading) to include the quality of studies and the likely levels of bias and applicability.

### Audit of protocols and guidelines

A protocol or a guideline which is not used is worthless – therefore regular audit is vital. This audit should be twofold, firstly establishing that the correct protocol or guideline is used and secondly that it is adhered to. Again the best-known protocols are related to the management of cardiac arrest. Most hospitals will audit performance at arrests and this may be compared to the protocols produced by the Resuscitation Council. Significant variation from their recommendations should be investigated and may highlight the need for further training.

### Litigation and protocols or guidelines

Unfortunately, litigation is also ubiquitous in modern society. In medical practice, failure to adhere to an established protocol or guideline may be taken as evidence of negligence. However, the reverse is not necessarily true – following a protocol or a guideline may not be a sufficient defence against allegations of negligence.

## Further reading

Agency for Health Care Policy and Research. *Acute Pain Management, Operative or Medical Procedures and Trauma*. Clinical Practice Guideline 92-0032. Rockville, Maryland, USA: Agency for Health Care Policy and Research Publications, 1992.

Harbour R, Miller J. A new system for grading recommendations in evidence based guidelines. *British Medical Journal* 2001; **323**: 334–336.

## Related topic of interest

Audit, p. 188.

# INDEX